THE
ULTIMATE AIP DIET COOKBOOK

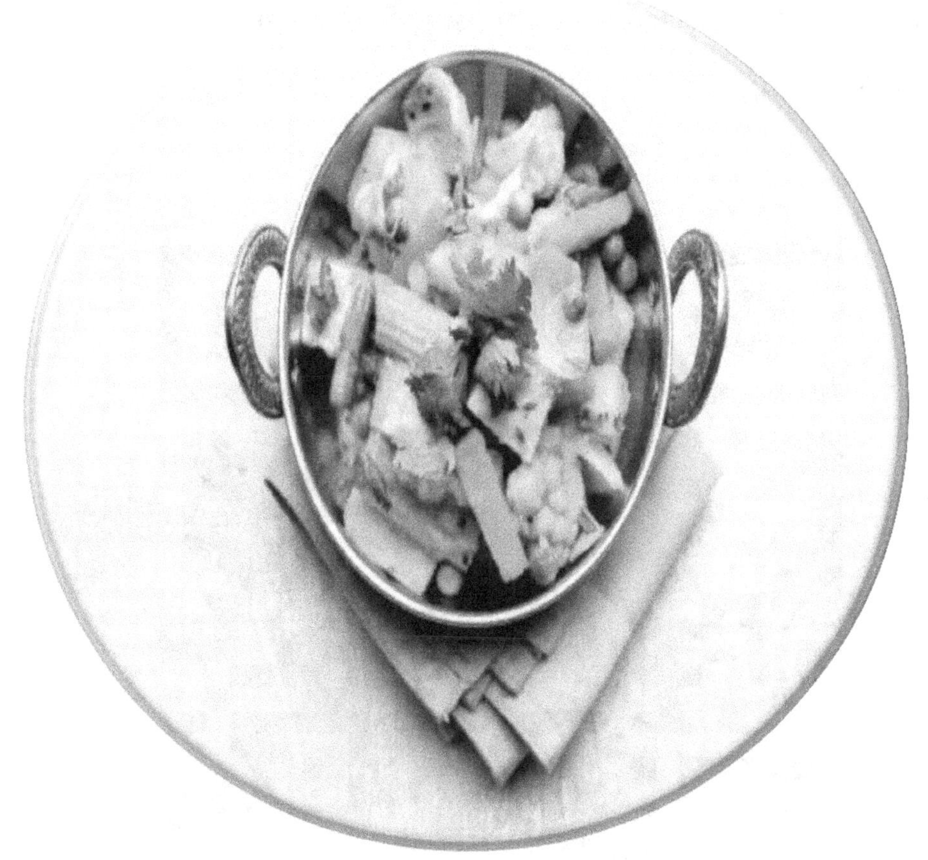

Restore Balance and Improve Your Health with Autoimmune Paleo Protocol

Dr. VIVIAN GREENE

Copyright © 2024 Dr. VIVIAN GREENE

Please scan the QR code to access additional books authored by Dr. Vivian Greene

Table of Contents

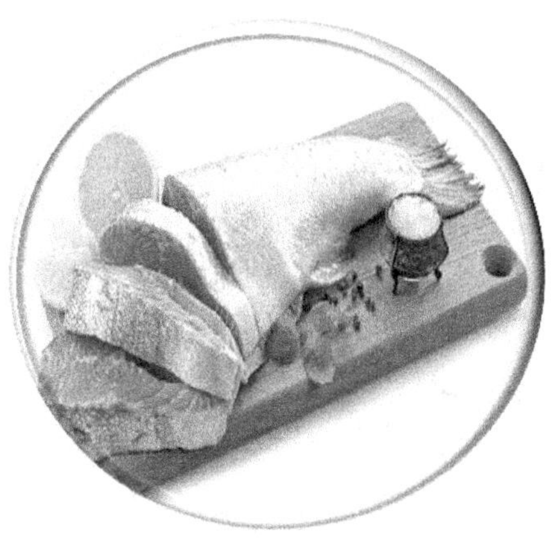

Introduction

We often go down several pathways in our quest for optimum health. While some bring clarity and vibrancy, others are meandering and filled with obstacles. Those who are struggling with the intricacies of autoimmune disorders might find hope in the Autoimmune Paleo Protocol (AIP) as they embark on this journey toward healing.

An in-depth discussion of the AIP diet—a revolutionary strategy intended to revitalize the body from the inside out—occurs inside the pages of this book. I've had the honor of seeing firsthand the significant effects of AIP on people dealing with autoimmune disorders as a writer committed to the science of health and well-being.

Understanding is the first step in every endeavor. The body's defensive mechanisms are interfered with by autoimmune illnesses, which cause the body to assault its tissues. The symptoms of this condition may seriously interfere with day-to-day functioning. Despite this, there is a chance to investigate the therapeutic value of food amid this difficulty.

Not just a food plan, the AIP protocol is a whole way of living designed to bring about internal balance. It is based on eliminating the things that cause inflammation and providing the body with meals that are high in nutrients and healing properties. AIP functions as a catalyst for healing and regeneration because of the careful component selection and thoughtful preparation.

Throughout these chapters, you will learn about the complexities of the AIP diet, from the principles to the finer points of cooking delicious, AIP-compliant meals. Every meal, from colorful breakfast bowls to enticing main courses and rich desserts, is a step toward regaining well-being in addition to being a gastronomic miracle.

But AIP affects all aspects of life, not just the kitchen. It develops a comprehensive approach to well-being and promotes stress management and mindful movement. There are powerful techniques to help you stay steady on your AIP path while managing social settings and eating out.

Not just a recipe book, this book is an empowering compendium that will help you find your equilibrium again, regain your energy, and change the way people think about health. It's evidence of the human body's tenacity and the significant influence that diet and lifestyle choices with awareness may have.

I welcome you to embrace the AIP lifestyle's guiding principles as well as the recipes as you set out on your adventure via the pages that follow. I hope that you will use this book as a compass to help you achieve a deep feeling of well-being, as well as restored health and vigor.

Understanding Autoimmune Conditions

Looking behind the scenes at the complicated defensive systems of the human body is necessary to comprehend autoimmune disorders. Protecting us against harmful substances like bacteria, viruses, and poisons is the job of our immune system, a biological engineering wonder. All too often, however, this system goes inward with autoimmune illnesses, mistaking bodily tissues for foes that need to be destroyed.

The symptoms of this constant attack on oneself might range from multiple sclerosis and celiac disease to lupus and rheumatoid arthritis. The immune system's erroneous reaction, which results in inflammation and tissue damage, is a commonality across these disorders. The end outcome is a wide range of symptoms that may affect almost every part of life, including stomach problems, joint discomfort, exhaustion, skin problems, and more.

The complex interactions between heredity, environment, and a dysregulated immune system must be understood to unravel the riddles behind autoimmune illnesses. Environmental factors often act as catalysts to awaken these circumstances; however, genetic predispositions might set the scene.

Stress, diseases, food, and even pollutants from the environment may all function as triggers. These stimuli cause the immune system to cascade into an inflammatory reaction, upsetting the delicate equilibrium in the body.

An increasing amount of studies indicate that gut health, molecular mimicry, and dysbiotic microbiota play a part in initiating and sustaining autoimmune illnesses, even if the exact etiology of these ailments is still unknown. An important part of immunological control is played by the gut, which is often referred to as the body's second brain. A leaky gut, a weakened intestinal lining, contributes to immune responses and exacerbates autoimmune reactions by allowing chemicals to enter the circulation.

The recognition of the significant influence that autoimmune disorders have on people goes beyond just understanding their processes. These disorders may have a profound impact on mental and emotional health in addition to their physical manifestations, upsetting everyday routines and testing the core of an individual's vitality.

The search for answers—new treatments, way of life adjustments, and dietary regimens such as the Autoimmune Paleo Protocol (AIP)—is fueled by this knowledge. Through understanding this complex interplay of immune dysregulation, environment, and genetics, we may take a step toward opening doors for treatment and, ideally, prevention.

We are on the verge of making progress in our understanding of autoimmune conditions. We hope to restore hope for a time when autoimmune conditions will not dictate an individual's quality of life by fusing scientific understanding with compassion and empowering people with the knowledge to navigate these challenging environments.

Overview of Autoimmune Paleo Protocol (AIP)

The Autoimmune Paleo Protocol (AIP) is a comprehensive dietary strategy intended to help people with autoimmune disorders manage their symptoms and recover. Building on the principles of the Paleo diet, the AIP adopts a stricter dietary approach by excluding extra items that are known to aggravate autoimmune responses and cause inflammation.

Fundamentally, the AIP emphasizes eliminating items that may cause inflammation, including grains, legumes, dairy products, processed sugars, plants that are related to nightshades, eggs, nuts, seeds, and certain spices. Reducing inflammation, promoting gut health, and halting more immune system activation are the goals of this elimination phase.

AIP stresses include nutrient-dense, therapeutic foods to feed the body at the same time. This comprises a diet rich in vegetables, lean meats, fish taken in the wild, avocado and coconut oil as healthy fats, and a modest amount of fruit. These nutrient-dense foods provide crucial vitamins, minerals, and antioxidants for a healthy immune system and general well-being.

Beyond only food adjustments, AIP promotes behavioral alterations. In addition to proper nutrition, stress reduction, restful sleep, moderate exercise, and creating a positive social circle are essential elements that enhance the AIP's holistic philosophy.

Usually, the procedure is broken up into two stages: the removal of trigger meals (elimination phase) and the assessment of each person's tolerance to certain foods (reintroduction phase). With the use of this individualized method, people may pinpoint the specific items that set them off, enabling them to design a diet that works for them.

AIP is a way of life that aims to balance the body again, quiet the immune system, and encourage internal healing. It is not only a band-aid solution. Following the Autoimmune Paleo Protocol's guidelines may lead to considerable improvements in symptoms and general well-being, but it also demands commitment and persistence as many people have reported.

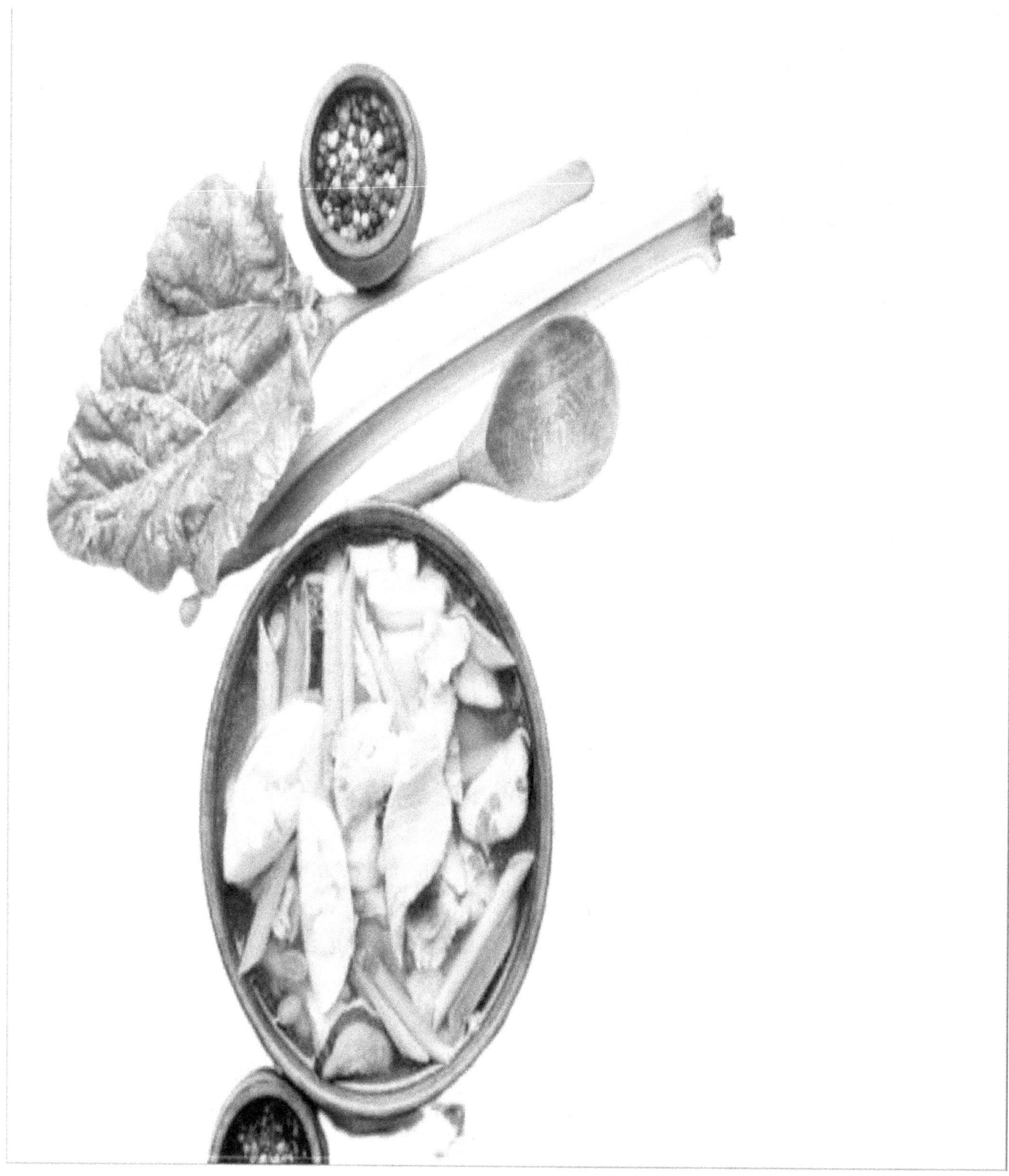

Chapter 1

What is the AIP Diet?

The Autoimmune Paleo Protocol (AIP) diet is a medical strategy designed especially for people with autoimmune diseases. It's a version of the Paleo diet, which is well-known for emphasizing whole, unadulterated meals. AIP, on the other hand, adopts a more focused strategy by excluding extra items that are shown to increase inflammatory responses and cause inflammation.

The main focus of the AIP diet is removing items that may cause inflammation. This entails cutting out nightshade vegetables (such as tomatoes, peppers, and eggplants), eggs, nuts, seeds, dairy products, processed sweets, and certain spices. These omissions are intended to lower inflammation, promote intestinal health, and stop the immune system from becoming more activated.

The AIP diet emphasizes nutrient-dense, therapeutic foods instead of these things that must be avoided. It promotes eating a variety of vegetables, particularly those high in phytonutrients and antioxidants. The cornerstones of this meal plan include premium meats, wild-caught fish, healthy fats from avocado and coconut oil, and a modest amount of fruits.

The main objective of the AIP diet is to repair the gut and reduce inflammation to reduce symptoms related to autoimmune disorders. The immune system is largely regulated by the gut, and autoimmune responses are thought to be exacerbated by a damaged gut lining, or leaky gut. The AIP diet seeks to balance the body by removing potentially toxic foods and adding ones that promote intestinal health.

Along with dietary changes, the AIP lifestyle promotes stress reduction methods, enough rest, moderate exercise, and creating a community of supportive people. These lifestyle elements support the AIP's holistic approach by balancing the food modifications.

The AIP diet usually consists of two stages: the elimination phase, during which trigger foods are eliminated, and the reintroduction phase, during which these foods are progressively added back to determine each person's tolerance. With the help of this individualized method, people may pinpoint certain trigger foods and develop a durable, individualized diet plan that promotes their general health and well-being.

Benefits of AIP for Autoimmune Conditions

For those suffering from autoimmune diseases, the Autoimmune Paleo Protocol (AIP) has several possible advantages, offering a comprehensive strategy that goes beyond simple symptom relief. The following are some noteworthy benefits of AIP for people with autoimmune conditions:

Cut Down on Inflammation:

The main goal of AIP is to avoid foods that are known to cause inflammation. As inflammation is often a major factor in autoimmune disorders, the goal of the AIP is to reduce inflammation by eliminating possible triggers such as nightshades, dairy, and wheat. Reducing inflammation may help with symptoms including weariness, joint discomfort, and skin problems.

Restoring Gut Health and Enhancing Digestive Health:

Through the elimination of items that may worsen leaky gut, a condition linked to autoimmune illnesses, the program places a priority on gut health. Stressing nutrient-dense, probiotic-rich, and gut-supportive meals may help repair the gut lining, which may lessen autoimmune reactions and enhance digestive health in general.

Recognizing Food Triggers:

Through the methodical reintroduction phase of the AIP, people may identify the precise foods that set off their autoimmune symptoms. With this individualized approach, people may create a diet that suits their requirements, which improves general health and symptom management.

Boosting Immune System and Nutrient Absorption:

The AIP's focus on nutrient-dense foods, such as vibrant veggies, premium meats, and healthy fats, supplies the vitamins, minerals, and antioxidants that the body needs to operate properly. This nutrient-dense diet helps the body absorb nutrients effectively, which may strengthen the immune system's resistance.

Increased Vitality and General Health:

When following the AIP diet, many people report feeling more energized, having a better mood, and feeling more general well-being. Through the management of underlying inflammation and the establishment of a more favorable intestinal environment, the AIP may facilitate a more lively and active way of living.

A Holistic Approach to Living:

In addition to food adjustments, the AIP promotes lifestyle adjustments such as stress reduction practices, getting enough sleep, and moderate exercise. These complementing elements help the body mend itself and make controlling autoimmune disorders a more all-encompassing strategy.

The AIP diet's emphasis on lowering inflammation, promoting gut health, and encouraging a nutrient-rich, customized diet is a viable option for those looking to manage their autoimmune diseases and enhance their quality of life, even if individual responses may differ.

How AIP Works: Understanding the Science

The Autoimmune Paleo Protocol (AIP) is based on a fundamental comprehension of the complex relationship—which is profoundly entwined in the domain of autoimmune disorders—between nutrition, inflammation, and the immune system.

Fundamentally, gut health and inflammation are the two main factors that are linked to autoimmune illnesses, and this is how AIP works. The following summarizes how the science behind AIP aids in the management of autoimmune conditions:

Cut Down on Inflammation:

An important cause of many autoimmune disorders is inflammation. AIP addresses this by removing foods that may cause inflammation and are known to activate immunological responses. The American Dietetic Plan (AIP) attempts to suppress the inflammatory cascade that leads to autoimmune symptoms including joint pain, exhaustion, and skin problems by eliminating culprits such as wheat, dairy, processed sweets, and nightshade vegetables.

Restoring Gut Health:

The emphasis on gut health is at the heart of the AIP methodology. The stomach, often called the body's "second brain," is essential for controlling the immune system. Leaky gut is a term used to describe a weakened intestinal lining that allows undigested particles to enter the circulation, inciting immunological reactions and perhaps aggravating autoimmune disorders. The goal of the AIP is to heal the gut lining, lower gut permeability, and lessen autoimmune triggers that come from the digestive system by emphasizing nutrient-dense, gut-healing foods.

Boosting Uptake of Nutrients:

The AIP diet's high nutritional content—which includes plenty of antioxidants, high-quality proteins, and colorful vegetables—supplies vital vitamins, minerals, and other nutrients that are critical for immune system performance. The AIP promotes adequate nutrition absorption by giving priority to nutrient-dense meals, which may strengthen the body's immunological response and resilience.

Phase of Personalized Reintroduction:

AIP includes a methodical reintroduction phase that enables people to progressively reintroduce items they have removed to determine their tolerance levels. Through the identification of certain trigger foods, this phase enables people to create a customized diet that maximizes nutritional variety while minimizing autoimmune responses.

A Comprehensive Strategy for Wellbeing:

Beyond only food adjustments, AIP promotes lifestyle adjustments including stress reduction, getting enough sleep, and moderate exercise. These lifestyle components support the food component and help create a more all-encompassing strategy for the management of autoimmune diseases.

Through a grasp of the science underpinning immune system regulation, gut health, and inflammation, the Autoimmune Paleo Protocol offers an organized approach to addressing the underlying causes of autoimmune illnesses. Its all-encompassing method seeks to balance the body again in addition to relieving symptoms, laying the groundwork for better health and well-being.

Chapter 2

Setting Up Your Kitchen for AIP

It takes planning to set up your kitchen for the Autoimmune Paleo Protocol (AIP) so that you have the equipment, supplies, and space needed to make AIP-compliant meals. Here's a guide to assist you in designing a kitchen that fits the AIP:

Eliminating Non-Complimentary Foods:

Take out any non-AIP goods from your cabinets, refrigerator, and pantry first. To make room for AIP-approved products, items such as grains, dairy, processed sugars, legumes, nightshade vegetables, eggs, nuts, and seeds should be given or put away.

AIP Pantry Essentials to Stock:

Stock your cupboard with items that align with the AIP to help you in your culinary ventures. This comprises:

- **Vegetables:** Beets, spinach, kale, broccoli, cauliflower, sweet potatoes, and carrots are among the fresh and frozen possibilities.
- **Wild-caught fish,** pastured poultry, and grass-fed meats are good sources of protein.
- **Avocado, coconut,** olive, and lard from pastured animals are examples of healthy fats.
- **AIP-friendly flours:** arrowroot powder, tapioca flour, and coconut flour for thickening and baking.
- **Herbs and Spices:** Herbs like garlic, ginger, turmeric, oregano, and rosemary are authorized by the American Paleopaths.

➢ Can goods include bone broth, coconut milk, and tinned fish (sardines or salmon).

➢ **Natural sweets:** AIP-approved sweets like as raw honey and maple syrup may be used in moderation.

Kitchen Utensils and Provisions:

Purchase kitchenware that makes AIP cooking easier:

➢ **Superior Blender:** Practical for blending sauces, purees, and smoothies.

➢ Convenient for making one-pot meals, stews, and soups that are AIP-compliant including slow cookers and instant pots.

➢ **Cutting boards and sharp knives** are necessary for slicing meat and vegetables.

➢ **Food processor:** Excellent for chopping vegetables and creating sauces from scratch.

➢ **Baking Sheets and Pans:** To meet the demands of AIP baking.

➢ **Storage Jars:** Ensure that the ingredients for your AIP are well-stocked and arranged.

Putting Your Kitchen in Order:

Organize your kitchen to facilitate smooth AIP cooking:

➢ **AIP Area Designated:** To avoid misunderstanding, set aside a certain area in your cupboards or pantry for AIP goods.

➢ **Organize Workspace:** To facilitate food preparation, keep worktops clear of clutter.

Supplies for Meal Preparation: Set aside containers for preparing meals in bulk and storing them.

Organizing Meals and Grocery Shopping:

Make grocery lists based on AIP recipes and plan your meals. This lessens the temptation to stray from the plan while grocery shopping and helps you make sure you have the required items.

A supportive atmosphere that makes AIP cooking simpler to follow and helps you start your path toward better health is created when your kitchen is organized according to the Autoimmune Paleo Protocol.

Stocking AIP Pantry Essentials

Stocking your pantry with essentials for the Autoimmune Paleo Protocol (AIP) lays the foundation for preparing delicious and compliant meals. Here's a comprehensive list of AIP-friendly pantry staples to keep on hand:

Vegetables:

- ➢ **Fresh and Frozen Options:** Spinach, kale, broccoli, cauliflower, sweet potatoes, carrots, beets, zucchini, squash, and any AIP-approved veggies based on your preferences.
- ➢ **Herbs and Greens:** Cilantro, parsley, basil, thyme, and any other fresh herbs for flavor.

Quality Proteins:

- ➢ **Grass-fed Meats:** Beef, lamb, and organ meats like liver or heart.
- ➢ **Pastured Poultry:** Chicken, turkey, and duck.
- ➢ **Wild-caught Fish:** Salmon, mackerel, cod, or any fish varieties compliant with AIP.

Healthy Fats:

- ➢ **Avocado Oil:** Great for cooking at higher temperatures.
- ➢ **Coconut Oil:** Ideal for baking and sautéing.
- ➢ **Olive Oil:** Perfect for dressings and low-heat cooking.
- ➢ **Lard or Tallow:** Rendered fat from pastured animals suitable for cooking.

AIP-friendly Flours and Starches:

➢ **Coconut Flour:** Used in baking and as a thickening agent.
➢ **Tapioca Flour:** Adds texture and used as a thickener.
➢ **Arrowroot Powder:** Another option for thickening sauces or baking.

Canned Goods:

➢ **Coconut Milk:** An essential ingredient for creamy sauces and soups.
➢ **Bone Broth:** A nutritious base for soups, stews, and sauces.
➢ **Canned Fish:** Salmon, sardines, or mackerel packed in water or olive oil.

Natural Sweeteners:

➢ **Raw Honey:** Use sparingly as a natural sweetener in moderation.
➢ **Maple Syrup:** Another option for sweetening AIP-approved recipes.

Herbs, Spices, and Seasonings:

➢ **Garlic Powder:** Adds flavor without the actual garlic.
➢ **Ginger:** Fresh or ground for its distinctive taste.
➢ **Turmeric:** Known for its anti-inflammatory properties.
➢ **Oregano, Rosemary, Thyme:** AIP-approved herbs to enhance flavor.

Miscellaneous:

➢ **Apple Cider Vinegar:** Used in dressings and marinades.
➢ **Coconut Aminos:** A soy-free alternative for seasoning and marinades.
➢ **Gelatin or Collagen Powder:** For added protein and gut health support.
➢ **AIP-friendly Snacks:** Dried fruits without added sugars, AIP-compliant jerky, or homemade snacks.

Storage:

➢ **Storage Containers:** Use to organize AIP ingredients and leftovers.
➢ **Mason Jars:** Great for storing homemade sauces, dressings, or bone broth.
➢ **Freezer Bags:** Handy for storing batch-cooked meals or extra portions.

By stocking your pantry with these AIP essentials, you'll have a well-equipped kitchen ready for preparing nourishing and compliant meals, making it easier to follow the Autoimmune Paleo Protocol and support your health goals.

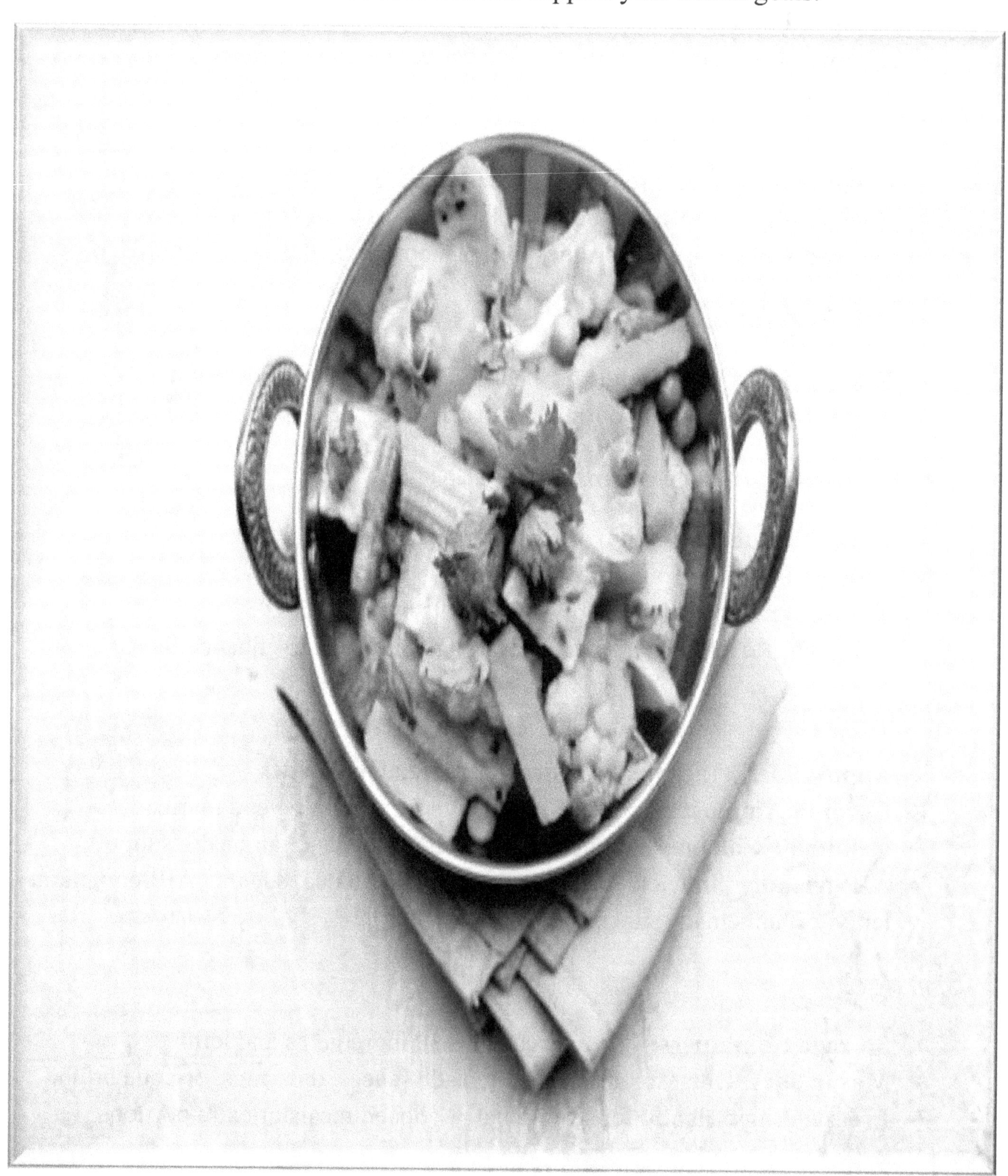

Meal Planning Tips and Strategies

Meal planning plays a pivotal role in successfully adhering to the Autoimmune Paleo Protocol (AIP). Here are some tips and strategies to help streamline your meal planning process:

Create a Weekly Meal Plan:

- **Set Aside Time:** Dedicate a specific time each week to plan your meals. Consider a day when you can comfortably browse recipes, create a shopping list, and prepare for the week ahead.
- **Variety and Balance:** Aim for variety in your meals to ensure a balanced intake of nutrients. Include diverse proteins, vegetables, and healthy fats to keep your meals interesting and nutritious.
- **Use AIP Recipes:** Explore AIP-specific cookbooks, websites, or resources to find recipes aligned with the protocol. Consider your preferences and dietary needs while selecting recipes.

Batch Cooking and Prepping:

- **Choose Batch-friendly Recipes:** Opt for recipes that can easily be batch-cooked or prepared in larger quantities. Soups, stews, and casseroles are excellent choices for batch cooking.
- **Prep Ingredients Ahead:** Wash, chop, and portion vegetables or meats in advance to streamline cooking during the week. Having prepped ingredients readily available can significantly reduce meal preparation time.

Grocery Shopping and List Making:

- **Make a Detailed Shopping List:** Based on your planned meals, create a comprehensive shopping list of AIP-approved ingredients. Organize the list by sections of the grocery store to expedite your shopping trip.
- **Stick to Your List:** While shopping, focus on purchasing items on your list to avoid impulse buys that might not align with the AIP guidelines.

Flexibility and Adaptability:

- ➤ **Be Flexible:** Life can be unpredictable, so allow room for flexibility in your meal plan. Have backup options or simple meals for days when time is limited or unexpected events arise.
- ➤ **Repurpose Leftovers:** Plan meals that can easily incorporate leftovers. For example, roast extra vegetables to use in salads or turn leftover protein into a stir-fry for the next day's meal.

Tracking and Evaluating:

- ➤ **Keep a Meal Planning Journal:** Track what worked well and what didn't in your meal plans. Note any favorite recipes, successful strategies, or adjustments needed for future planning.
- ➤ **Evaluate and Adjust:** Regularly assess the effectiveness of your meal plans. Adjust recipes, shopping habits, or cooking strategies based on your experiences to optimize your meal planning process.

Plan for Success:

- ➤ **Stay Organized:** Use meal planning apps, calendars, or printable templates to stay organized and keep track of your plans.
- ➤ **Celebrate Success:** Acknowledge and celebrate your accomplishments in sticking to your meal plan. Recognizing your progress can help maintain motivation and consistency.

By implementing these meal planning tips and strategies, you can streamline your AIP journey, make healthier food choices, and simplify the process of preparing nourishing and compliant meals aligned with the Autoimmune Paleo Protocol.

Chapter 3

DELICIOUS AIP RECIPES FOR BREAKFAST

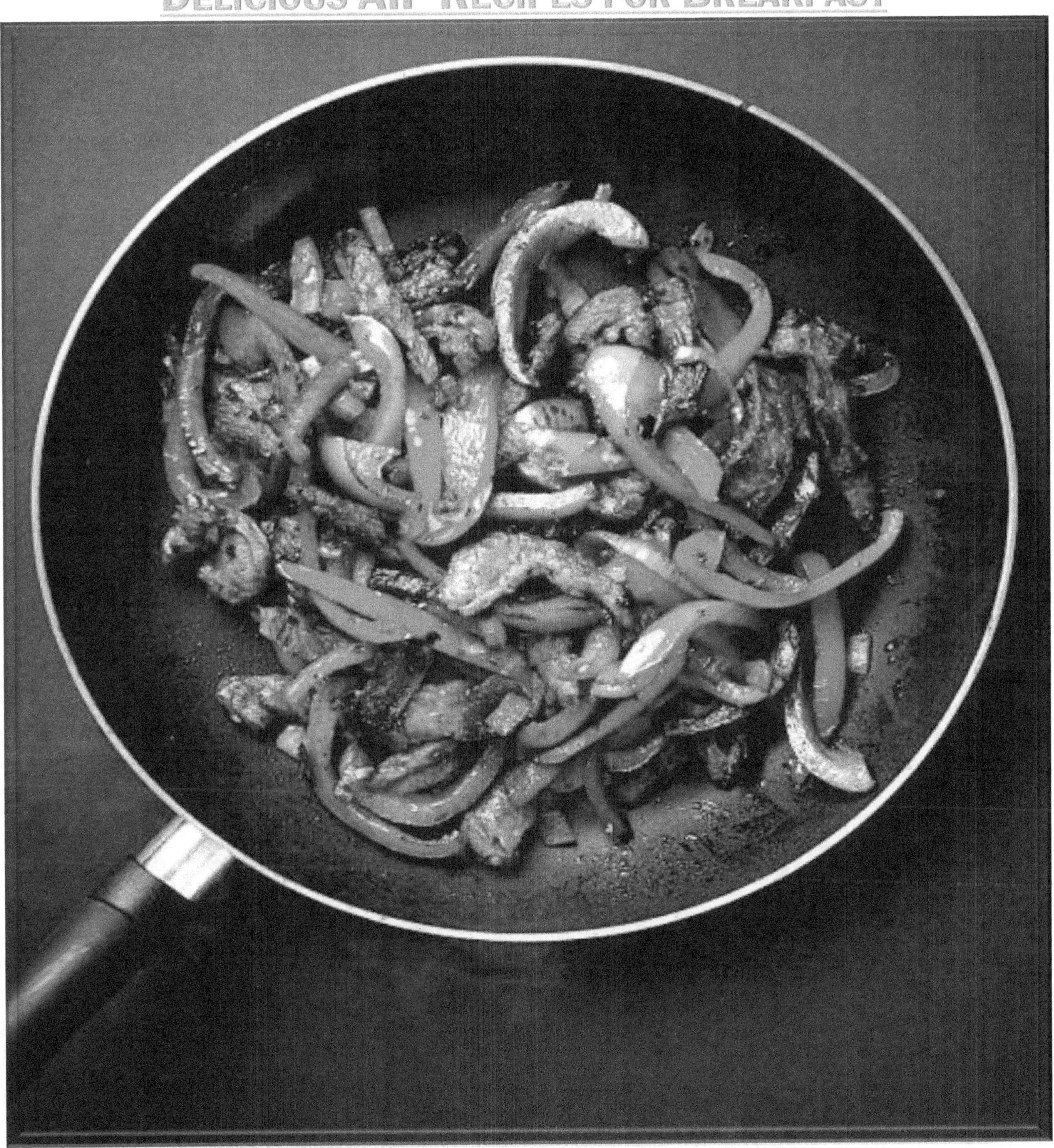

Sweet Potato and Kale Breakfast Bowl

INGREDIENTS:

1. 1 medium sweet potato, cubed
2. 1 cup kale, chopped
3. 2 slices bacon, cooked and crumbled
4. 1 tablespoon coconut oil
5. Salt and pepper to taste

INSTRUCTIONS:

1. In a skillet, heat coconut oil over medium heat.
2. Add sweet potato cubes and sauté until tender, about 8-10 minutes.
3. Add chopped kale and cook until wilted.
4. Season with salt and pepper.
5. Serve in a bowl, topped with crumbled bacon.

Nutrition per Serving:
- *Calories: 280*
- *Protein: 8g*
- *Carbohydrates: 25g*
- *Fat: 17g*

Berry Coconut Breakfast Bowl

INGREDIENTS:

1. 1 cup mixed berries (blueberries, raspberries, strawberries)
2. 1/2 cup shredded coconut
3. 1 tablespoon chia seeds
4. Coconut milk (as needed for desired consistency)

INSTRUCTIONS:

1. Blend mixed berries and coconut milk until smooth.
2. Pour the berry mixture into a bowl.
3. Top with shredded coconut and chia seeds.

Nutrition per Serving:

- ❖ Calories: 220
- ❖ Protein: 3g
- ❖ Carbohydrates: 20g
- ❖ Fat: 15g

Turkey and Plantain Breakfast Bowl

INGREDIENTS:

1. 1 ripe plantain, sliced
2. 4 ounces cooked turkey, shredded
3. 1 cup spinach
4. 1 tablespoon avocado oil

INSTRUCTIONS:

1. Heat avocado oil in a pan over medium heat.
2. Sauté plantain slices until golden brown.
3. Add shredded turkey and spinach, cooking until spinach wilts.
4. Serve in a bowl.

Nutrition per Serving:

- Calories: 310
- Protein: 22g
- Carbohydrates: 28g
- Fat: 14g

Pumpkin Pie Breakfast Bowl

INGREDIENTS:

1. 1/2 cup pumpkin puree
2. 1/4 cup coconut cream
3. 1 tablespoon maple syrup (optional)
4. 1/2 teaspoon cinnamon
5. 1/4 teaspoon nutmeg
6. Chopped walnuts for topping

INSTRUCTIONS:

1. Mix pumpkin puree, coconut cream, maple syrup (if using), and spices.
2. Heat in the microwave or on the stove until warm.
3. Top with chopped walnuts.

Nutrition per Serving:

❖ Calories: 220
❖ Protein: 3g
❖ Carbohydrates: 20g
❖ Fat: 15g

Chicken and Vegetable Breakfast Bowl

INGREDIENTS:

1. 4 ounces cooked chicken, diced
2. 1 cup cauliflower rice
3. 1/2 cup sliced mushrooms
4. 1/4 cup diced bell peppers
5. 1 tablespoon olive oil
6. Salt and herbs for seasoning

INSTRUCTIONS:

1. Sauté cauliflower rice, mushrooms, and bell peppers in olive oil until tender.
2. Add diced chicken and cook until heated through.
3. Season with salt and herbs.
4. Serve in a bowl.

Nutrition per Serving:

❖ Calories: 280
❖ Protein: 25g
❖ Carbohydrates: 10g
❖ Fat: 15g

Apple Cinnamon Breakfast Bowl

INGREDIENTS:

1. 1 apple, diced
2. 2 tablespoons coconut flakes
3. 1 tablespoon raisins
4. 1/2 teaspoon cinnamon
5. 1/4 teaspoon vanilla extract

INSTRUCTIONS:

1. In a saucepan, simmer diced apple with a splash of water until soft.
2. Stir in coconut flakes, raisins, cinnamon, and vanilla extract.
3. Cook until flavors combine and the mixture thickens.
4. Serve in a bowl.

Nutrition per Serving:

❖ Calories: 180
❖ Protein: 1g
❖ Carbohydrates: 30g
❖ Fat: 8g

Beef and Spinach Breakfast Bowl

INGREDIENTS:

1. 4 ounces cooked ground beef
2. 1 cup spinach leaves
3. 1/2 avocado, sliced
4. 1 tablespoon olive oil
5. Salt and pepper to taste

INSTRUCTIONS:

1. In a skillet, heat olive oil over medium heat.
2. Add spinach and cook until wilted.
3. Place cooked ground beef and spinach in a bowl.
4. Top with sliced avocado.
5. Season with salt and pepper.

Nutrition per Serving:

❖ Calories: 350
❖ Protein: 22g
❖ Carbohydrates: 10g
❖ Fat: 25g

Mango Tango Breakfast Bowl

INGREDIENTS:

1. 1 ripe mango, diced
2. 1/4 cup sliced strawberries
3. 1 tablespoon shredded coconut
4. Lime zest for garnish

INSTRUCTIONS:

1. Mix diced mango and sliced strawberries in a bowl.
2. Sprinkle with shredded coconut and lime zest.
3. Serve chilled.

Nutrition per Serving:

❖ Calories: 190
❖ Protein: 2g
❖ Carbohydrates: 45g
❖ Fat: 2g

Shrimp and Zucchini Breakfast Bowl

INGREDIENTS:

1. 4 ounces cooked shrimp
2. 1 zucchini, spiralized
3. 1/4 cup chopped tomatoes
4. 1 tablespoon chopped basil
5. 1 tablespoon lemon juice

INSTRUCTIONS:

1. Sauté spiralized zucchini in a pan until tender.
2. Add cooked shrimp, chopped tomatoes, and chopped basil.
3. Cook for a few minutes until heated through.
4. Drizzle with lemon juice before serving.

Nutrition per Serving:

- ❖ Calories: 220
- ❖ Protein: 25g
- ❖ Carbohydrates: 12g
- ❖ Fat: 8g

Blueberry Banana Breakfast Bowl

INGREDIENTS:

1. 1 ripe banana, mashed
2. 1/2 cup blueberries
3. 2 tablespoons shredded coconut
4. 1 tablespoon chopped almonds

INSTRUCTIONS:

1. Mash the banana in a bowl.
2. Top with blueberries, shredded coconut, and chopped almonds.
3. Enjoy as is or slightly warmed.

Nutrition per Serving:

❖ Calories: 250
❖ Protein: 3g
❖ Carbohydrates: 40g
❖ Fat: 10g

Nutrient-Packed Smoothies and Shakes

Berry Blast Smoothie

INGREDIENTS:

1. 1 cup mixed berries (strawberries, blueberries, raspberries)
2. 1 ripe banana (frozen)
3. 1 cup coconut milk
4. 1 tablespoon collagen powder
5. 1 teaspoon honey (optional)

INSTRUCTIONS:

1. Blend all ingredients until smooth.
2. Add more coconut milk for desired consistency.
3. Serve chilled.

Nutrition per Serving:

❖ Calories: 210 | Protein: 6g | Fat: 11g | Carbohydrates: 26g | Fiber: 6g

Tropical Paradise Shake

INGREDIENTS:

1. 1 cup diced pineapple
2. 1 ripe mango
3. 1 cup coconut water
4. 1 tablespoon chia seeds
5. 1/2 teaspoon grated ginger

INSTRUCTIONS:

1. Blend all ingredients until well combined.
2. Adjust consistency with additional coconut water if needed.
3. Enjoy cold.

Nutrition per Serving:

❖ Calories: 220 | Protein: 3g | Fat: 2g | Carbohydrates: 54g | Fiber: 8g

Green Vitality Smoothie

INGREDIENTS:

1. 2 cups spinach
2. 1/2 avocado
3. 1 green apple, cored and chopped
4. 1 cup coconut water
5. Juice of 1 lime

INSTRUCTIONS:

1. Blend spinach and coconut water until smooth.
2. Add remaining ingredients and blend until creamy.
3. Serve chilled.

Nutrition per Serving:

❖ Calories: 230 | Protein: 4g | Fat: 11g | Carbohydrates: 32g | Fiber: 11g

Creamy Banana Almond Shake

INGREDIENTS:

1. 2 ripe bananas (frozen)
2. 2 tablespoons almond butter
3. 1 1/2 cups almond milk
4. 1 teaspoon cinnamon
5. Pinch of sea salt

INSTRUCTIONS:

1. Blend bananas, almond butter, and almond milk until creamy.
2. Add cinnamon and salt, blend again.
3. Serve immediately.

Nutrition per Serving:

❖ Calories: 320 | Protein: 7g | Fat: 18g | Carbohydrates: 38g | Fiber: 7g

Orange Carrot Revitalizer

INGREDIENTS:

1. 2 oranges, peeled
2. 1 large carrot, chopped
3. 1/2 cup coconut water
4. 1 tablespoon honey (optional)
5. Ice cubes (as desired)

INSTRUCTIONS:

1. Blend oranges, carrot, and coconut water until smooth.
2. Add honey if desired, blend again.
3. Serve over ice.

Nutrition per Serving:

❖ Calories: 180 | Protein: 3g | Fat: 1g | Carbohydrates: 45g | Fiber: 8g

Blueberry Spinach Power Smoothie

INGREDIENTS:

1. 1 cup frozen blueberries
2. 2 cups spinach
3. 1 ripe banana
4. 1 cup coconut milk
5. 1 tablespoon hemp seeds

INSTRUCTIONS:

1. Blend blueberries, spinach, banana, and coconut milk until creamy.
2. Add hemp seeds, blend briefly.
3. Enjoy immediately.

Nutrition per Serving:

❖ Calories: 270 | Protein: 6g | Fat: 12g | Carbohydrates: 38g | Fiber: 10g

Pineapple Ginger Refresher

INGREDIENTS:

1. 1 cup diced pineapple
2. 1-inch piece of fresh ginger, peeled
3. 1 cup coconut water
4. Juice of 1 lime
5. Mint leaves for garnish

INSTRUCTIONS:

1. Blend pineapple, ginger, coconut water, and lime juice until smooth.
2. Pour into glasses and garnish with mint leaves.
3. Serve chilled.

Nutrition per Serving:

❖ Calories: 160 | Protein: 2g | Fat: 1g | Carbohydrates: 40g | Fiber: 4g

Creamy Coconut Avocado Shake

INGREDIENTS:

1. 1 ripe avocado
2. 1/2 cup coconut cream
3. 1 tablespoon shredded coconut
4. 1 1/2 cups coconut water
5. 1 teaspoon vanilla extract

INSTRUCTIONS:

1. Blend avocado, coconut cream, shredded coconut, and coconut water until creamy.
2. Add vanilla extract, blend again.
3. Serve with a sprinkle of shredded coconut on top.

Nutrition per Serving:

❖ Calories: 300 | Protein: 3g | Fat: 27g | Carbohydrates: 18g | Fiber: 10g

Kiwi Lime Detox Smoothie

INGREDIENTS:

1. 2 kiwis, peeled and sliced
2. Juice of 2 limes
3. 1 cup cucumber, chopped
4. 1 cup coconut water
5. 1 tablespoon fresh mint leaves

INSTRUCTIONS:

1. Blend kiwis, lime juice, cucumber, and coconut water until well combined.
2. Add mint leaves and blend for a few seconds.
3. Pour into glasses and serve cold.

Nutrition per Serving:

❖ Calories: 150 | Protein: 3g | Fat: 1g | Carbohydrates: 35g | Fiber: 8g

Mixed Berry Coconut Shake

INGREDIENTS:

1. 1 cup mixed berries (blackberries, raspberries)
2. 1/2 cup full-fat coconut milk
3. 1 tablespoon shredded coconut
4. 1 tablespoon collagen powder
5. Ice cubes (as desired)

INSTRUCTIONS:

1. Blend mixed berries, coconut milk, shredded coconut, and collagen powder until smooth.
2. Add ice cubes and blend again for a frosty texture.
3. Serve immediately.

Nutrition per Serving:

❖ Calories: 240 | Protein: 6g | Fat: 15g | Carbohydrates: 22g | Fiber: 8g

Creative AIP Pancake and Waffle Alternatives

Coconut Flour Pancakes

INGREDIENTS:

1. 1/4 cup coconut flour
2. 4 eggs
3. 1/4 cup coconut milk
4. 1/2 teaspoon baking soda
5. 1 tablespoon coconut oil (for cooking)

INSTRUCTIONS:

1. Whisk eggs in a bowl, then add coconut flour, coconut milk, and baking soda. Mix until smooth.
2. Heat coconut oil in a pan over medium heat. Pour small circles of batter onto the pan.
3. Cook for 2-3 minutes until bubbles form, then flip and cook for another 1-2 minutes.

Nutrition per Serving:

❖ Calories: 180
❖ Protein: 8g
❖ Fat: 11g
❖ Carbohydrates: 11g
❖ Fiber: 6g

Tigernut Flour Waffles

INGREDIENTS:

1. 1 cup tigernut flour
2. 2 tablespoons coconut oil (melted)
3. 3/4 cup coconut milk
4. 1 teaspoon baking soda

INSTRUCTIONS:

1. Mix tigernut flour, melted coconut oil, coconut milk, and baking soda until well combined.
2. Preheat waffle iron and lightly grease with coconut oil. Pour batter onto the iron and cook according to the manufacturer's instructions.

Nutrition per Serving:

❖ Calories: 220
❖ Protein: 4g
❖ Fat: 15g
❖ Carbohydrates: 20g
❖ Fiber: 8g

Cassava Flour Pancakes

INGREDIENTS:

1. 1 cup cassava flour
2. 2 eggs
3. 1/2 cup coconut milk
4. 1 teaspoon baking powder (AIP compliant)
5. 2 tablespoons maple syrup (optional)

INSTRUCTIONS:

1. Mix cassava flour, eggs, coconut milk, baking powder, and maple syrup (if using) until smooth.
2. Heat a skillet over medium heat, pour batter, and cook for 2-3 minutes on each side.

Nutrition per Serving:

❖ Calories: 240
❖ Protein: 5g
❖ Fat: 7g
❖ Carbohydrates: 40g
❖ Fiber: 2g

Plantain Waffles

INGREDIENTS:

1. 2 ripe plantains
2. 2 tablespoons coconut flour
3. 2 tablespoons coconut oil
4. 1 teaspoon vanilla extract (AIP compliant)
5. Pinch of salt

INSTRUCTIONS:

1. Blend peeled plantains, coconut flour, coconut oil, vanilla extract, and salt until smooth.
2. Pour batter into a preheated waffle iron and cook until golden brown.

Nutrition per Serving:

❖ Calories: 180
❖ Protein: 2g
❖ Fat: 7g
❖ Carbohydrates: 30g
❖ Fiber: 3g

Pumpkin Pancakes

INGREDIENTS:

1. 1 cup canned pumpkin puree
2. 2 tablespoons coconut flour
3. 2 eggs
4. 1 teaspoon cinnamon
5. 1/2 teaspoon baking soda

INSTRUCTIONS:

1. Mix pumpkin puree, coconut flour, eggs, cinnamon, and baking soda until well combined.
2. Heat a skillet over medium heat, pour batter, and cook for 2-3 minutes on each side.

Nutrition per Serving:

- Calories: 160
- Protein: 8g
- Fat: 6g
- Carbohydrates: 20g
- Fiber: 8g

Banana Flour Waffles

INGREDIENTS:

1. 1 cup banana flour
2. 2 eggs
3. 1/2 cup coconut milk
4. 1 tablespoon coconut oil
5. 1 teaspoon baking powder (AIP compliant)

INSTRUCTIONS:

1. Mix banana flour, eggs, coconut milk, coconut oil, and baking powder until smooth.
2. Preheat waffle iron and cook batter according to the manufacturer's instructions.

Nutrition per Serving:

- ❖ Calories: 200
- ❖ Protein: 5g
- ❖ Fat: 8g
- ❖ Carbohydrates: 30g
- ❖ Fiber: 5g

Sweet Potato Pancakes

INGREDIENTS:

1. 1 cup mashed sweet potato
2. 2 tablespoons coconut flour
3. 2 eggs
4. 1/2 teaspoon cinnamon
5. Pinch of salt

INSTRUCTIONS:

1. Mix mashed sweet potato, coconut flour, eggs, cinnamon, and salt until thoroughly combined.
2. Heat a skillet over medium heat, pour batter, and cook for 2-3 minutes on each side.

Nutrition per Serving:

❖ Calories: 160
❖ Protein: 6g
❖ Fat: 4g
❖ Carbohydrates: 25g
❖ Fiber: 5g

Arrowroot Flour Waffles

INGREDIENTS:

1. 1 cup arrowroot flour
2. 2 eggs
3. 1/2 cup coconut milk
4. 2 tablespoons coconut oil
5. 1 teaspoon apple cider vinegar

INSTRUCTIONS:

1. Mix arrowroot flour, eggs, coconut milk, coconut oil, and apple cider vinegar until well combined.
2. Preheat waffle iron and cook batter according to the manufacturer's instructions.

Nutrition per Serving:

❖ Calories: 190
❖ Protein: 4g
❖ Fat: 9g
❖ Carbohydrates: 25g
❖ Fiber: 1g

Acorn Squash Pancakes

INGREDIENTS:

1. 1 cup cooked and mashed acorn squash
2. 2 tablespoons coconut flour
3. 2 eggs
4. 1/2 teaspoon vanilla extract (AIP compliant)
5. Pinch of cinnamon

INSTRUCTIONS:

1. Combine mashed acorn squash, coconut flour, eggs, vanilla extract, and cinnamon until well blended.
2. Heat a skillet over medium heat, pour batter, and cook for 2-3 minutes on each side.

Nutrition per Serving:

- Calories: 140
- Protein: 7g
- Fat: 4g
- Carbohydrates: 20g
- Fiber: 6g

Cauliflower Waffles

INGREDIENTS:

1. 2 cups riced cauliflower (cooked and drained)
2. 2 tablespoons coconut flour
3. 2 eggs
4. 1/2 teaspoon garlic powder
5. Salt and pepper to taste

INSTRUCTIONS:

1. Mix cooked and drained riced cauliflower, coconut flour, eggs, garlic powder, salt, and pepper until combined.
2. Preheat waffle iron and cook batter according to the manufacturer's instructions

Nutrition per Serving:

❖ Calories: 160
❖ Protein: 8g
❖ Fat: 6g
❖ Carbohydrates: 20g
❖ Fiber: 8g

Chapter 4

Satisfying Soups, Salads, and Appetizers

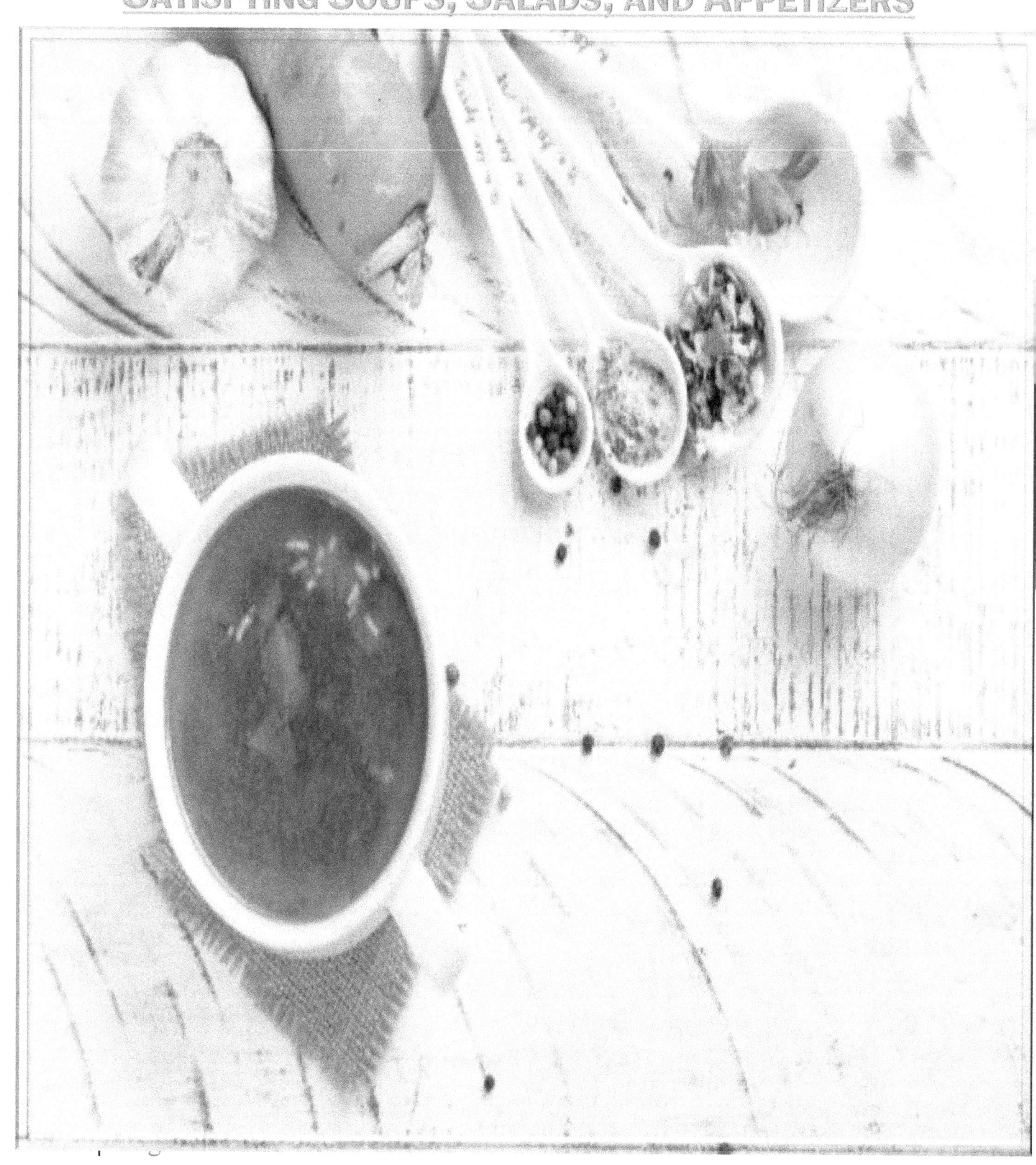

Healing Bone Broth Soup

INGREDIENTS:

1. 4 cups bone broth
2. 1 cup shredded chicken
3. 2 cups chopped carrots
4. 1 cup chopped celery
5. 1 tablespoon chopped fresh parsley
6. Salt to taste

INSTRUCTIONS:

1. In a pot, bring bone broth to a gentle simmer.
2. Add shredded chicken, carrots, and celery.
3. Simmer for 15-20 minutes until vegetables are tender.
4. Season with salt and garnish with fresh parsley.

Nutrition per Serving:

- Calories: 150
- Protein: 18g
- Fat: 4g
- Carbohydrates: 10g
- Fiber: 2g

Butternut Squash & Apple Soup

INGREDIENTS:

1. 1 butternut squash, peeled and diced
2. 2 apples, peeled and chopped
3. 1 onion, chopped
4. 4 cups bone broth
5. 1 teaspoon ground cinnamon
6. Salt and pepper to taste

INSTRUCTIONS:

1. In a pot, sauté onions until translucent.
2. Add butternut squash, apples, bone broth, and cinnamon.
3. Simmer for 20-25 minutes until squash is tender.
4. Blend until smooth, season with salt and pepper.

Nutrition per Serving:

❖ Calories: 180
❖ Protein: 3g
❖ Fat: 1g
❖ Carbohydrates: 45g
❖ Fiber: 8g

Nourishing Chicken Vegetable Soup

INGREDIENTS:

1. 4 cups chicken broth
2. 2 cups shredded chicken
3. 1 cup diced carrots
4. 1 cup diced zucchini
5. 1 cup chopped spinach
6. 2 garlic cloves, minced
7. Salt and herbs to taste

INSTRUCTIONS:

1. In a pot, bring chicken broth to a boil.
2. Add shredded chicken, carrots, zucchini, garlic, and simmer for 15 minutes.
3. Add chopped spinach, cook for an additional 5 minutes.
4. Season with salt and herbs before serving.

Nutrition per Serving:

❖ Calories: 220
❖ Protein: 25g
❖ Fat: 3g
❖ Carbohydrates: 15g
❖ Fiber: 4g

Turmeric Infused Vegetable Soup

INGREDIENTS:

1. 4 cups vegetable broth
2. 2 cups diced sweet potatoes
3. 1 cup chopped broccoli
4. 1 cup sliced carrots
5. 1 teaspoon turmeric powder
6. Salt and pepper to taste

INSTRUCTIONS:

1. In a pot, bring vegetable broth to a boil.
2. Add sweet potatoes, broccoli, carrots, and turmeric.
3. Simmer for 15-20 minutes until vegetables are tender.
4. Season with salt and pepper before serving.

Nutrition per Serving:

❖ Calories: 170
❖ Protein: 3g
❖ Fat: 0g
❖ Carbohydrates: 40g
❖ Fiber: 8g

Creamy Coconut and Cauliflower Soup

INGREDIENTS:

1. 1 head cauliflower, chopped
2. 1 can coconut milk
3. 3 cups chicken or vegetable broth
4. 2 garlic cloves, minced
5. 1 teaspoon ground ginger
6. Salt to taste

INSTRUCTIONS:

1. In a pot, combine cauliflower, coconut milk, broth, garlic, and ginger.
2. Bring to a boil, then reduce heat and simmer for 20 minutes.
3. Blend until smooth using an immersion blender or regular blender.
4. Season with salt and serve.

Nutrition per Serving:

❖ Calories: 180
❖ Protein: 5g
❖ Fat: 15g
❖ Carbohydrates: 10g
❖ Fiber: 4g

Zesty Carrot and Ginger Soup

INGREDIENTS:

1. 6 large carrots, chopped
2. 1 onion, chopped
3. 3 cups bone broth
4. 2 tablespoons grated ginger
5. Zest and juice of 1 orange
6. Salt and pepper to taste

INSTRUCTIONS:

1. Sauté onions until soft, then add carrots, bone broth, ginger, and orange zest.
2. Bring to a boil, then simmer for 20-25 minutes until carrots are tender.
3. Blend the soup until smooth, add orange juice, and season with salt and pepper.

Nutrition per Serving:

❖ Calories: 140
❖ Protein: 4g
❖ Fat: 1g
❖ Carbohydrates: 30g
❖ Fiber: 7g

Savory Spinach and Chicken Soup

INGREDIENTS:

1. 4 cups chicken broth
2. 2 cups shredded chicken
3. 2 cups chopped spinach
4. 1 onion, diced
5. 2 garlic cloves, minced
6. 1 tablespoon fresh lemon juice
7. Salt and herbs to taste

INSTRUCTIONS:

1. In a pot, sauté onions and garlic until softened.
2. Add chicken broth, shredded chicken, and chopped spinach.
3. Simmer for 10-15 minutes until flavors meld.
4. Stir in fresh lemon juice, season with salt and herbs before serving.

Nutrition per Serving:

❖ Calories: 180
❖ Protein: 20g
❖ Fat: 4g
❖ Carbohydrates: 8g
❖ Fiber: 2g

Celeriac and Leek Soup

INGREDIENTS:

1. 2 leeks, sliced
2. 1 celeriac bulb, peeled and diced
3. 4 cups bone broth
4. 2 tablespoons coconut oil
5. 1 teaspoon dried thyme
6. Salt and pepper to taste

INSTRUCTIONS:

1. Sauté leeks in coconut oil until tender.
2. Add diced celeriac, bone broth, and dried thyme.
3. Simmer for 20-25 minutes until celeriac is soft.
4. Blend the soup until smooth, season with salt and pepper.

Nutrition per Serving:

❖ Calories: 160
❖ Protein: 6g
❖ Fat: 8g
❖ Carbohydrates: 20g
❖ Fiber: 4g

Pumpkin and Ginger Soup

INGREDIENTS:

1. 2 cups pumpkin puree
2. 3 cups chicken or vegetable broth
3. 1 tablespoon grated fresh ginger
4. 1 onion, chopped
5. 1 tablespoon coconut oil
6. Salt and cinnamon to taste

INSTRUCTIONS:

1. Sauté onions in coconut oil until translucent.
2. Add pumpkin puree, broth, grated ginger, and bring to a simmer.
3. Cook for 15-20 minutes, then blend until smooth.
4. Season with salt and a sprinkle of cinnamon before serving.

Nutrition per Serving:

❖ Calories: 120
❖ Protein: 3g
❖ Fat: 6g
❖ Carbohydrates: 15g
❖ Fiber: 4g

Beet and Carrot Detox Soup

INGREDIENTS:

1. 2 beets, peeled and chopped
2. 3 carrots, chopped
3. 1 onion, diced
4. 4 cups vegetable broth
5. 2 tablespoons apple cider vinegar
6. Salt and fresh herbs to taste

INSTRUCTIONS:

1. Sauté onions until softened.
2. Add beets, carrots, vegetable broth, and apple cider vinegar.
3. Simmer for 20-25 minutes until vegetables are tender.
4. Blend the soup until smooth, season with salt and herbs.

Nutrition per Serving:

- ❖ Calories: 140
- ❖ Protein: 3g
- ❖ Fat: 0g
- ❖ Carbohydrates: 30g
- ❖ Fiber: 8g

Citrus Avocado Salad

INGREDIENTS:

1. 1 ripe avocado, sliced
2. 1 grapefruit, segmented
3. Mixed greens
4. 2 tbsp olive oil
5. 1 tbsp fresh lemon juice
6. Salt and pepper to taste

INSTRUCTIONS:

1. Toss mixed greens with olive oil, lemon juice, salt, and pepper.
2. Arrange avocado slices and grapefruit segments on top.
3. Serve immediately.

Nutrition per Serving:

- Calories: 220
- Fat: 18g
- Carbohydrates: 15g
- Fiber: 9g
- Protein: 3g

Strawberry Spinach Salad

INGREDIENTS:

1. 2 cups spinach leaves
2. 1 cup sliced strawberries
3. ¼ cup sliced red onion
4. 2 tbsp balsamic vinegar
5. 1 tbsp olive oil
6. Salt and pepper to taste

INSTRUCTIONS:

1. Combine spinach, strawberries, and red onion in a bowl.
2. Drizzle with balsamic vinegar and olive oil.
3. Season with salt and pepper, toss well, and serve.

Nutrition per Serving:

❖ Fat: 7g
❖ Carbohydrates: 11g
❖ Fiber: 4g
❖ Protein: 2g

Tuna Cucumber Salad

INGREDIENTS:

1. 1 can (5 oz) tuna, drained
2. 1 cucumber, thinly sliced
3. 1 cup cherry tomatoes, halved
4. Fresh parsley, chopped
5. 2 tbsp lemon juice
6. 2 tbsp olive oil
7. Salt and pepper to taste

INSTRUCTIONS:

1. Mix tuna, cucumber, and cherry tomatoes in a bowl.
2. Drizzle with lemon juice and olive oil.
3. Season with salt, pepper, and garnish with parsley before scrving.

Nutrition per Serving:

❖ Calories: 240
❖ Fat: 15g
❖ Carbohydrates: 9g
❖ Fiber: 3g
❖ Protein: 20g

Roasted Beet and Arugula Salad

INGREDIENTS:

1. 2 medium beets, roasted and sliced
2. 2 cups arugula
3. ¼ cup toasted pumpkin seeds
4. 2 tbsp apple cider vinegar
5. 1 tbsp olive oil
6. Salt and pepper to taste

INSTRUCTIONS:

1. Arrange arugula on a plate, top with roasted beets and pumpkin seeds.
2. Drizzle with apple cider vinegar and olive oil.
3. Season with salt and pepper, then serve.

Nutrition per Serving:

❖ Calories: 160
❖ Fat: 9g
❖ Carbohydrates: 16g
❖ Fiber: 6g
❖ Protein: 5g

Berry Coconut Breakfast Bowl

INGREDIENTS:

5. 1 cup mixed berries (blueberries, raspberries, strawberries)
6. 1/2 cup shredded coconut
7. 1 tablespoon chia seeds
8. Coconut milk (as needed for desired consistency)

INSTRUCTIONS:

4. Blend mixed berries and coconut milk until smooth.
5. Pour the berry mixture into a bowl.
6. Top with shredded coconut and chia seeds.

Nutrition per Serving:

❖ Calories: 220
❖ Protein: 3g
❖ Carbohydrates: 20g
❖ Fat: 15g

Mango Chicken Salad

INGREDIENTS:

1. 2 cups cooked chicken, shredded
2. 1 ripe mango, diced
3. 1 cup cucumber, diced
4. 2 green onions, chopped
5. Juice of 1 lime
6. 2 tbsp coconut aminos
7. Fresh cilantro for garnish

INSTRUCTIONS:

1. In a bowl, mix chicken, mango, cucumber, and green onions.
2. Add lime juice and coconut aminos, toss gently.
3. Garnish with cilantro before serving.

Nutrition per Serving:

❖ Fat: 5g
❖ Carbohydrates: 25g
❖ Fiber: 4g
❖ Protein: 30g

Shrimp and Pineapple Salad

INGREDIENTS:

1. 1 lb shrimp, cooked and peeled
2. 1 cup diced pineapple
3. 1 red bell pepper, thinly sliced
4. 2 cups mixed greens
5. 2 tbsp fresh lime juice
6. 1 tbsp olive oil
7. Salt and pepper to taste

INSTRUCTIONS:

1. Combine shrimp, pineapple, bell pepper, and mixed greens.
2. Drizzle with lime juice and olive oil.
3. Season with salt and pepper, toss well, and serve.

Nutrition per Serving:

- Calories: 220
- Fat: 7g
- Carbohydrates: 18g
- Fiber: 3g
- Protein: 24g

Zesty Tuna and Olive Salad

INGREDIENTS:

1. 2 cans (5 oz each) tuna, drained
2. ½ cup sliced black olives
3. ½ cup chopped cucumber
4. 2 tbsp chopped fresh parsley
5. 2 tbsp apple cider vinegar
6. 2 tbsp extra virgin olive oil
7. Salt and pepper to taste

INSTRUCTIONS:

1. Mix tuna, black olives, cucumber, and parsley in a bowl.
2. Drizzle with apple cider vinegar and olive oil.
3. Season with salt and pepper, toss gently, and serve.

Nutrition per Serving:

❖ Calories: 290
❖ Fat: 18g
❖ Carbohydrates: 3g
❖ Fiber: 1g
❖ Protein: 30g

Radicchio and Orange Salad

INGREDIENTS:

1. 1 head radicchio, thinly sliced
2. 2 oranges, segmented
3. ¼ cup sliced red onion
4. 2 tbsp balsamic vinegar
5. 2 tbsp avocado oil
6. Salt and pepper to taste

INSTRUCTIONS:

1. Combine radicchio, orange segments, and red onion in a bowl.
2. Drizzle with balsamic vinegar and avocado oil.
3. Season with salt and pepper, toss gently, and serve.

Nutrition per Serving:

❖ Calories: 150
❖ Fat: 9g
❖ Carbohydrates: 18g
❖ Fiber: 5g
❖ Protein: 2g

Turkey and Cranberry Salad

INGREDIENTS:

1. 2 cups cooked turkey, diced
2. ½ cup chopped celery
3. ¼ cup dried cranberries
4. 2 tbsp chopped fresh sage
5. 2 tbsp lemon juice
6. 2 tbsp coconut cream
7. Salt and pepper to taste

INSTRUCTIONS:

1. Mix turkey, celery, cranberries, and sage in a bowl.
2. In a separate bowl, whisk together lemon juice and coconut cream.
3. Pour the dressing over the salad, season with salt and pepper, and mix well.

Nutrition per Serving:

- ❖ Calories: 220
- ❖ Fat: 5g
- ❖ Carbohydrates: 14g
- ❖ Fiber: 2g
- ❖ Protein: 30g

Summer Berry Spinach Salad

INGREDIENTS:

1. 2 cups baby spinach
2. ½ cup mixed berries (blueberries, raspberries, strawberries)
3. ¼ cup sliced almonds (if tolerated)
4. 2 tbsp balsamic vinegar
5. 1 tbsp olive oil
6. Salt and pepper to taste

INSTRUCTIONS:

1. Combine spinach, mixed berries, and sliced almonds in a bowl.
2. Drizzle with balsamic vinegar and olive oil.
3. Season with salt and pepper, toss gently, and serve.

Nutrition per Serving:

- Calories: 160
- Fat: 10g
- Carbohydrates: 14g
- Fiber: 6g
- Protein: 4g

AIP Veggie Skewers

INGREDIENTS:

1. Zucchini, sliced
2. Carrots, cut into chunks
3. Bell peppers, diced
4. Red onion, cut into wedges
5. Fresh parsley, chopped (for garnish)

INSTRUCTIONS:

1. Preheat grill or grill pan over medium heat.
2. Thread vegetables onto skewers.
3. Grill skewers for 8-10 minutes, turning occasionally until veggies are tender.
4. Garnish with chopped parsley and serve.

Nutrition per Serving:

❖ Calories: 45
❖ Carbohydrates: 10g
❖ Fiber: 3g
❖ Protein: 1g
❖ Fat: 0g

Guacamole Stuffed Endive Leaves

INGREDIENTS:

1. Ripe avocados
2. Fresh lime juice
3. Garlic powder
4. Salt
5. Endive leaves

INSTRUCTIONS:

1. Mash avocados with lime juice, garlic powder, and salt to taste.
2. Spoon guacamole into endive leaves.
3. Arrange on a platter and serve.

Nutrition per Serving:

❖ Calories: 60
❖ Carbohydrates: 4g
❖ Fiber: 3g
❖ Protein: 1g
❖ Fat: 5g

AIP Bacon-Wrapped Dates

INGREDIENTS:

1. Medjool dates, pitted
2. Bacon slices (nitrate-free)
3. Toothpicks

INSTRUCTIONS:

1. Preheat oven to 375°F (190°C).
2. Wrap each date with a strip of bacon and secure with a toothpick.
3. Place on a baking sheet and bake for 15-18 minutes until bacon is crispy.
4. Serve warm.

Nutrition per Serving:

❖ Calories: 120
❖ Carbohydrates: 18g
❖ Fiber: 2g
❖ Protein: 3g
❖ Fat: 5g

AIP Tuna Salad Cucumber Bites

INGREDIENTS:

1. Cucumbers, sliced into rounds
2. Canned tuna (in olive oil or water)
3. Avocado, mashed
4. Red onion, finely diced
5. Fresh parsley, chopped

INSTRUCTIONS:

1. In a bowl, mix tuna, mashed avocado, diced red onion, chopped parsley, and lemon juice.
2. Place a spoonful of tuna salad onto each cucumber slice.
3. Season with a pinch of salt and pepper if desired.
4. Arrange on a platter and serve.

Nutrition per Serving:

- Calories: 70
- Carbohydrates: 3g
- Fiber: 2g
- Protein: 7g
- Fat: 3g

AIP Stuffed Mushrooms

INGREDIENTS:

1. Mushrooms, cleaned and stems removed
2. Ground turkey or chicken
3. Onion, finely chopped
4. Garlic, minced
5. Fresh thyme, chopped
6. Avocado oil
7. Salt

INSTRUCTIONS:

1. Preheat oven to 375°F (190°C).
2. In a skillet, sauté onion and garlic in avocado oil until softened.
3. Add ground meat and cook until browned.
4. Stir in chopped thyme and season with salt.
5. Stuff mushroom caps with the meat mixture.
6. Place on a baking sheet and bake for 15-18 minutes.
7. Serve warm.

Nutrition per Serving:
- Calories: 90
- Carbohydrates: 3g
- Fiber: 1g
- Protein: 12g
- Fat: 4gFat: 15g

AIP Coconut Shrimp

INGREDIENTS:

1. Large shrimp, peeled and deveined
2. Coconut flour
3. Unsweetened shredded coconut
4. AIP-friendly seasoning blend
5. Avocado oil for frying

INSTRUCTIONS:

1. Coat shrimp in coconut flour seasoned with AIP-friendly spices.
2. Dip coated shrimp in beaten egg (optional) and then roll in shredded coconut.
3. Heat avocado oil in a skillet over medium-high heat.
4. Fry shrimp until golden brown and crispy, about 2-3 minutes per side.
5. Drain on a paper towel and serve with a dipping sauce if desired.

Nutrition per Serving:

- Calories: 130
- Carbohydrates: 5g
- Fiber: 2g
- Protein: 10g
- Fat: 7g

AIP Sweet Potato Bites

INGREDIENTS:

1. Sweet potatoes, peeled and sliced into rounds
2. Cooked shredded chicken
3. Avocado, mashed
4. Red cabbage, thinly sliced
5. Fresh cilantro, chopped
6. Lime juice
7. Salt

INSTRUCTIONS:

1. Preheat oven to 400°F (200°C).
2. Roast sweet potato rounds on a baking sheet for 20-25 minutes until tender.
3. In a bowl, mix shredded chicken, mashed avocado, sliced cabbage, chopped cilantro, lime juice, and a pinch of salt.
4. Top each sweet potato round with the chicken-avocado mixture.
5. Serve warm.

Nutrition per Serving:

❖ Calories: 90
❖ Carbohydrates: 10g
❖ Fiber: 2g
❖ Protein: 6g
❖ Fat: 3g

AIP Herb-Crusted Chicken Tenders

INGREDIENTS:

1. Chicken breast, cut into strips
2. Fresh parsley, chopped
3. Fresh thyme, chopped
4. Garlic powder
5. Onion powder
6. Avocado oil
7. Salt

INSTRUCTIONS:

1.
2. Preheat oven to 375°F (190°C).
3. Mix chopped herbs, garlic powder, onion powder, and salt on a plate.
4. Coat chicken strips with avocado oil and then dredge in the herb mixture.
5. Place chicken on a baking sheet lined with parchment paper.
6. Bake for 20-25 minutes until chicken is cooked through and golden brown.
7. Serve with AIP-friendly dipping sauce if desired.

Nutrition per Serving:

- ❖ Calories: 150
- ❖ Carbohydrates: 1g
- ❖ Fiber: 0g
- ❖ Protein: 25g
- ❖ Fat: 5g

AIP Deviled Eggs

INGREDIENTS:

1. Hard-boiled eggs, peeled
2. Avocado, mashed
3. Dijon mustard (AIP-friendly)
4. Fresh chives, chopped
5. Salt and pepper (optional)

INSTRUCTIONS:

1. Cut hard-boiled eggs in half lengthwise and remove yolks.
2. In a bowl, mix mashed avocado, Dijon mustard, chopped chives, and salt (and pepper if tolerated) with egg yolks until smooth.
3. Spoon or pipe the avocado mixture into the egg white halves.
4. Garnish with additional chopped chives.
5. Serve chilled.

Nutrition per Serving:

❖ Calories: 90
❖ Carbohydrates: 2g
❖ Fiber: 1g
❖ Protein: 6g
❖ Fat: 7g

Chapter 5

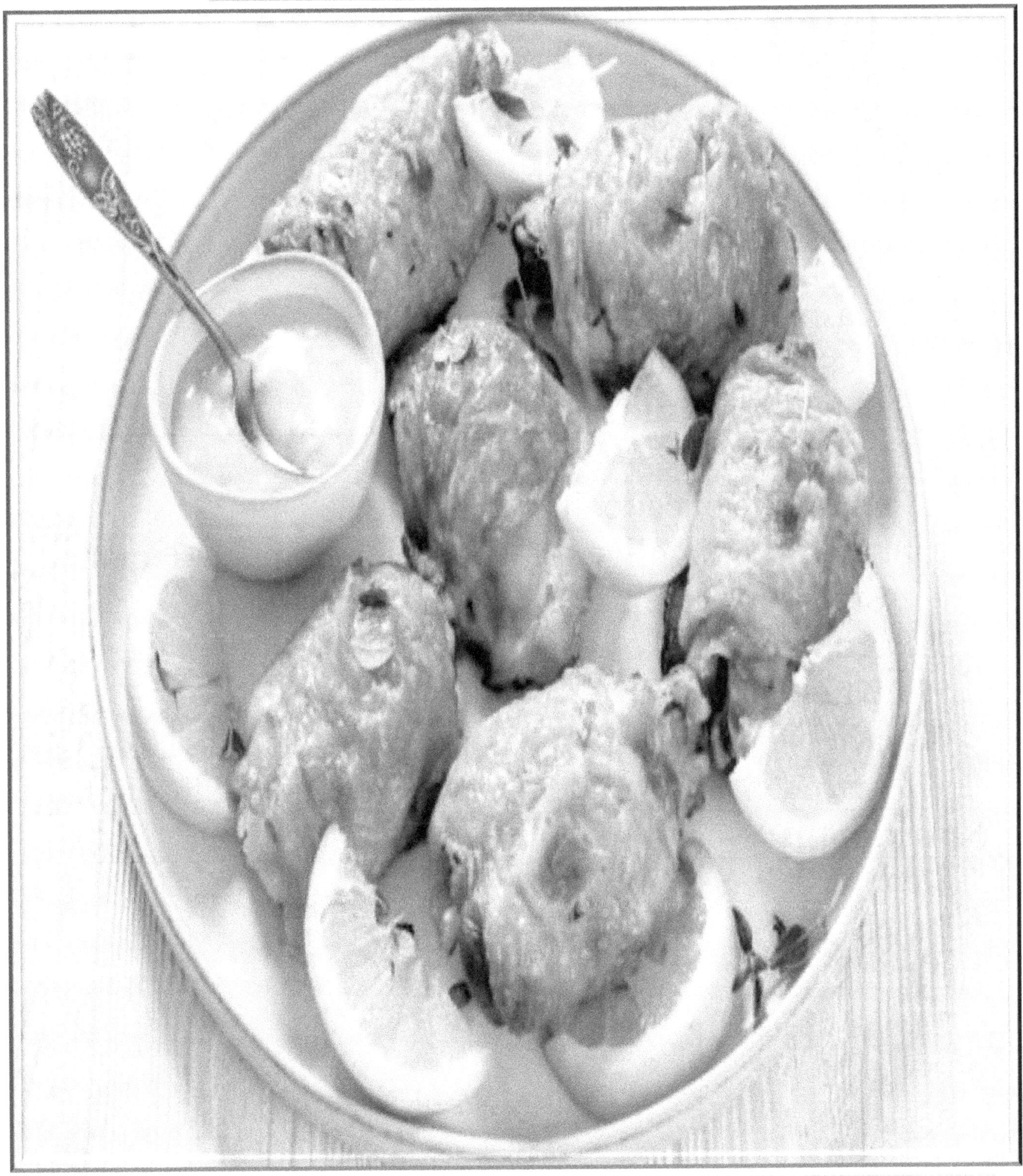

Lemon Herb Roasted Chicken Thighs

INGREDIENTS:

1. 4 bone-in, skin-on chicken thighs
2. 2 tablespoons olive oil
3. 2 cloves garlic, minced
4. 1 tablespoon fresh lemon juice
5. 1 teaspoon lemon zest
6. 1 teaspoon dried thyme
7. 1 teaspoon dried rosemary
8. Salt and pepper to taste

INSTRUCTIONS:

1. Preheat the oven to 400°F (200°C).
2. In a bowl, mix olive oil, garlic, lemon juice, lemon zest, thyme, rosemary, salt, and pepper.
3. Pat dry the chicken thighs and rub them with the herb mixture.
4. Place the chicken on a baking sheet and roast for 30-35 minutes until golden brown and cooked through.

Nutrition per Serving:

❖ Calories: 280

❖ Protein: 25g

❖ Fat: 18g

❖ Carbohydrates: 1g

❖ Fiber: 0g

❖ Sugars: 0g

AIP Turkey and Vegetable Stir-Fry

INGREDIENTS:

1. 1 pound turkey breast, thinly sliced
2. 2 tablespoons coconut aminos
3. 2 tablespoons apple cider vinegar
4. 2 tablespoons coconut oil
5. 2 cloves garlic, minced
6. 1-inch fresh ginger, grated
7. 2 cups broccoli florets
8. 1 red bell pepper, sliced
9. Salt to taste
10. Chopped green onions for garnish

INSTRUCTIONS:

1. In a bowl, marinate turkey slices with coconut aminos and apple cider vinegar for 15-20 minutes.
2. Heat coconut oil in a skillet over medium-high heat. Add garlic and ginger, sauté for 1 minute.
3. Add marinated turkey and cook until browned.
4. Add broccoli and bell pepper, cook until vegetables are tender yet crisp.
5. Season with salt, garnish with green onions, and serve.

Nutrition per Serving:

- ❖ Calories: 290
- ❖ Protein: 28g
- ❖ Fat: 12g
- ❖ Carbohydrates: 10g
- ❖ Fiber: 3g
- ❖ Sugars: 5g

Herbed Grilled Chicken Skewers

INGREDIENTS:

1. 1 pound chicken breast, cut into cubes
2. 2 tablespoons olive oil
3. 2 tablespoons chopped fresh basil
4. 1 tablespoon chopped fresh parsley
5. 1 tablespoon chopped fresh mint
6. 1 teaspoon garlic powder
7. Salt and pepper to taste

INSTRUCTIONS:

1. In a bowl, combine olive oil, chopped herbs, garlic powder, salt, and pepper.
2. Marinate chicken cubes in the herb mixture for at least 30 minutes.
3. Thread the marinated chicken onto skewers.
4. Grill over medium heat for 8-10 minutes, turning occasionally, until chicken is cooked through.

Nutrition per Serving:

❖ Calories: 220
❖ Protein: 30g
❖ Fat: 9g
❖ Carbohydrates: 1g
❖ Fiber: 0g
❖ Sugars: 0g

Coconut-Crusted Chicken Tenders

INGREDIENTS:

1. 1 pound chicken tenders
2. 1 cup shredded unsweetened coconut
3. 2 tablespoons coconut flour
4. 1 teaspoon garlic powder
5. 1 teaspoon onion powder
6. 1/2 teaspoon sea salt
7. 2 eggs, beaten
8. Avocado oil for frying

INSTRUCTIONS:

1. Preheat oven to 400°F (200°C).
2. In a bowl, mix shredded coconut, coconut flour, garlic powder, onion powder, and salt.
3. Dip chicken tenders in beaten eggs, then coat with the coconut mixture.
4. Heat avocado oil in a skillet over medium heat. Fry chicken tenders until golden brown, about 2-3 minutes per side.
5. Transfer chicken to a baking sheet and bake for 10-15 minutes until cooked through.

Nutrition per Serving:

❖ Calories: 280
❖ Protein: 25g
❖ Fat: 17g
❖ Carbohydrates: 6g
❖ Fiber: 4g
❖ Sugars: 2g

Herbed Turkey Meatballs

INGREDIENTS:

1. 1 pound ground turkey
2. 1/4 cup chopped fresh parsley
3. 2 tablespoons chopped fresh basil
4. 1 tablespoon chopped fresh oregano
5. 2 cloves garlic, minced
6. 1 teaspoon onion powder
7. 1/2 teaspoon sea salt
8. 1/4 teaspoon black pepper (optional, omit for AIP)

INSTRUCTIONS:

1. Preheat oven to 375°F (190°C).
2. In a bowl, combine ground turkey, chopped herbs, garlic, onion powder, salt, and pepper.
3. Shape the mixture into meatballs and place them on a baking sheet lined with parchment paper.
4. Bake for 20-25 minutes until the meatballs are cooked through.

Nutrition per Serving:

❖ Calories: 180
❖ Protein: 22g
❖ Fat: 9g
❖ Carbohydrates: 2g
❖ Fiber: 0g
❖ Sugars: 0g

AIP Chicken Zoodle Soup

INGREDIENTS:

1. 2 tablespoons coconut oil
2. 1 onion, diced
3. 2 carrots, sliced
4. 2 cclcry stalks, sliced
5. 2 cloves garlic, minced
6. 6 cups chicken bone broth
7. 2 cups shredded cooked chicken
8. 2 zucchinis, spiralized into noodles
9. 2 tablespoons chopped fresh parsley
10. Salt and pepper to taste

INSTRUCTIONS:

1. In a pot, heat coconut oil over medium heat. Add onion, carrots, celery, and garlic. Sauté until softened.
2. Pour in chicken bone broth and bring to a boil. Reduce heat and simmer for 15-20 minutes.
3. Add shredded chicken and zucchini noodles. Cook for an additional 5-7 minutes until zoodles are tender.
4. Season with salt, pepper, and garnish with fresh parsley before serving.

Nutrition per Serving:

- Calories: 180
- Protein: 20g
- Fat: 8g
- Carbohydrates: 7g
- Fiber: 2g
- Sugars: 3g

Garlic Herb Baked Turkey Breast

INGREDIENTS:

1. 1 boneless turkey breast
2. 3 tablespoons olive oil
3. 4 cloves garlic, minced
4. 1 tablespoon chopped fresh rosemary
5. 1 tablespoon chopped fresh thyme
6. 1 teaspoon sea salt
7. 1/2 teaspoon black pepper (optional, omit for AIP)

INSTRUCTIONS:

1. Preheat oven to 375°F (190°C).
2. In a bowl, mix olive oil, minced garlic, chopped rosemary, thyme, salt, and pepper (if using).
3. Place the turkey breast in a baking dish and rub it with the herb mixture.
4. Bake for 45-55 minutes until the internal temperature reaches 165°F (74°C). Let it rest before slicing.

Nutrition per Serving:

❖ Calories: 220
❖ Protein: 30g
❖ Fat: 10g
❖ Carbohydrates: 1g
❖ Fiber: 0g
❖ Sugars: 0g

Chicken and Veggie Sheet Pan Dinner

INGREDIENTS:

1. 4 boneless chicken breasts
2. 2 cups Brussels sprouts, halved
3. 2 cups cubed butternut squash
4. 1 red onion, sliced
5. 2 tablespoons balsamic vinegar
6. 3 tablespoons olive oil
7. 2 cloves garlic, minced
8. 1 teaspoon dried thyme
9. Salt and pepper to taste

INSTRUCTIONS:

1. Preheat oven to 400°F (200°C).
2. Place chicken breasts, Brussels sprouts, butternut squash, and red onion on a sheet pan.
3. In a bowl, whisk together balsamic vinegar, olive oil, minced garlic, dried thyme, salt, and pepper.
4. Drizzle the mixture over the chicken and vegetables. Toss to coat evenly.
5. Roast for 25-30 minutes until chicken is cooked through and vegetables are tender.

Nutrition per Serving:

- ❖ Calories: 320
- ❖ Protein: 28g
- ❖ Fat: 15g
- ❖ Carbohydrates: 18g
- ❖ Fiber: 6g
- ❖ Sugars: 6g

Lemon Garlic Turkey Cutlets

INGREDIENTS:

1. 1 pound turkey cutlets
2. 2 tablespoons arrowroot powder
3. 2 tablespoons coconut oil
4. 3 cloves garlic, minced
5. 1/4 cup chicken broth
6. 2 tablespoons fresh lemon juice
7. Zest of 1 lemon
8. 1 tablespoon chopped fresh parsley
9. Salt and pepper to taste

INSTRUCTIONS:

1. Coat turkey cutlets with arrowroot powder, salt, and pepper.
2. Heat coconut oil in a skillet over medium-high heat. Cook turkey cutlets until golden brown on both sides, about 3-4 minutes per side. Remove from skillet and set aside.
3. In the same skillet, add minced garlic and cook for 1 minute. Pour in chicken broth, lemon juice, and lemon zest. Bring to a simmer.
4. Return turkey cutlets to the skillet. Simmer for 3-4 minutes until the sauce thickens and turkey is cooked through.
7. Garnish with chopped parsley before serving.

Nutrition per Serving:

❖ Calories: 240

❖ Protein: 30g

❖ Fat: 11g

❖ Carbohydrates: 6g

❖ Fiber: 1g

❖ Sugars: 1g

AIP Chicken Curry with Cauliflower Rice

INGREDIENTS:

1. 1 pound boneless chicken thighs, cubed
2. 1 tablespoon coconut oil
3. 1 onion, diced
4. 3 cloves garlic, minced
5. 1 tablespoon grated fresh ginger
6. 2 teaspoons turmeric powder
7. 1 teaspoon ground coriander
8. 1 teaspoon ground cumin (optional, omit for AIP)
9. 1 can (13.5 oz) coconut milk
10. 2 cups cauliflower rice
11. Fresh cilantro for garnish
12. Salt to taste

INSTRUCTIONS:

1. In a skillet, heat coconut oil over medium heat. Sauté diced onion, garlic, and ginger until softened.
2. Add cubed chicken and cook until browned.
3. Stir in turmeric, ground coriander, and ground cumin (if using). Cook for 1 minute.
4. Pour in coconut milk, bring to a simmer, and cook for 10-15 minutes until chicken is cooked through and the sauce thickens.
5. In a separate pan, sauté cauliflower rice until tender.
6. Serve the chicken curry over cauliflower rice, garnish with fresh cilantro.

Nutrition per Serving:

❖ Calories: 320
❖ Protein: 22g
❖ Fat: 25g
❖ Carbohydrates: 8g
❖ Fiber: 3g
❖ Sugars: 3g

Baked Lemon Herb Salmon

INGREDIENTS:

1. 4 salmon fillets
2. 2 tablespoons olive oil
3. 2 tablespoons fresh lemon juice
4. 2 cloves garlic, minced
5. 1 teaspoon dried thyme
6. Salt and pepper (omit pepper for AIP)

INSTRUCTIONS:

1. Preheat oven to 375°F (190°C).
2. In a bowl, mix olive oil, lemon juice, minced garlic, thyme, salt, and pepper.
3. Place salmon fillets on a baking sheet. Coat each fillet with the lemon herb mixture.
4. Bake for 15-20 minutes until salmon is cooked through

Nutrition per Serving:

❖ Calories: 280
❖ Protein: 30g
❖ Fat: 16g
❖ Carbohydrates: 2g

AIP Garlic Shrimp Stir-Fry

INGREDIENTS:

1. 1 pound shrimp, peeled and deveined
2. 2 tablespoons coconut aminos
3. 2 tablespoons coconut oil
4. 3 cloves garlic, minced
5. 1 cup sliced bell peppers
6. 1 cup broccoli florets
7. Salt to taste

INSTRUCTIONS:

1. Heat coconut oil in a skillet over medium heat. Add minced garlic and sauté until fragrant.
2. Add shrimp and stir until they start turning pink.
3. Stir in coconut aminos, bell peppers, and broccoli. Cook until vegetables are tender.
4. Season with salt and serve.

Nutrition per Serving:

- ❖ Calories: 250
- ❖ Protein: 24g
- ❖ Fat: 12g
- ❖ Carbohydrates: 8g

Grilled Herb Marinated Swordfish

INGREDIENTS:

1. 4 swordfish steaks
2. ¼ cup olive oil
3. 2 tablespoons fresh parsley, chopped
4. 2 tablespoons fresh cilantro, chopped
5. 2 cloves garlic, minced
6. 1 teaspoon lemon zest
7. Salt to taste

INSTRUCTIONS:

1. In a bowl, mix olive oil, parsley, cilantro, minced garlic, lemon zest, and salt.
2. Coat swordfish steaks with the herb marinade. Let it sit for 20-30 minutes.
3. Preheat grill to medium-high heat. Grill swordfish for 4-5 minutes per side or until cooked through.

Nutrition per Serving (5 oz):

❖ Calories: 320
❖ Protein: 30g
❖ Fat: 20g
❖ Carbohydrates: 1g

AIP Baked Lemon Garlic Cod

INGREDIENTS:

1. 4 cod fillets
2. 3 tablespoons olive oil
3. 2 tablespoons fresh lemon juice
4. 2 cloves garlic, minced
5. 1 teaspoon dried oregano
6. Salt to taste

INSTRUCTIONS:

1. Preheat oven to 375°F (190°C).
2. In a bowl, combine olive oil, lemon juice, minced garlic, dried oregano, and salt.
3. Place cod fillets in a baking dish and pour the lemon garlic mixture over them.
4. Bake for 20-25 minutes or until the cod flakes easily with a fork.

Nutrition per Serving:

❖ Calories: 180
❖ Protein: 25g
❖ Fat: 8g
❖ Carbohydrates: 1g

AIP Cilantro Lime Shrimp Salad

INGREDIENTS:

1. 1 pound cooked shrimp, peeled
2. 1 cup chopped cucumber
3. 1 cup cherry tomatoes, halved
4. ¼ cup chopped fresh cilantro
5. 2 tablespoons olive oil
6. 2 tablespoons fresh lime juice
7. Salt to taste

INSTRUCTIONS:

1. In a bowl, combine cooked shrimp, chopped cucumber, cherry tomatoes, and cilantro.
2. Drizzle olive oil and lime juice over the salad. Mix well.
3. Season with salt and refrigerate for 30 minutes before serving.

Nutrition per Serving (6 oz):

❖ Calories: 220
❖ Protein: 30g
❖ Fat: 10g
❖ Carbohydrates: 6g

AIP Baked Herb Crusted Halibut

INGREDIENTS:

1. 4 halibut fillets
2. ¼ cup coconut flour
3. 2 tablespoons chopped fresh parsley
4. 2 tablespoons chopped fresh basil
5. 2 tablespoons coconut oil, melted
6. Salt to taste

INSTRUCTIONS:

1. Preheat oven to 400°F (200°C).
2. In a bowl, mix coconut flour, chopped parsley, chopped basil, and salt.
3. Coat halibut fillets with melted coconut oil, then coat with the herb mixture.
4. Place fillets on a baking sheet and bake for 12-15 minutes until fish is cooked through.

Nutrition per Serving:

❖ Calories: 260
❖ Protein: 30g
❖ Fat: 12g
❖ Carbohydrates: 6g

AIP Tuna Cakes

INGREDIENTS:

1. 2 cans (5 oz each) tuna, drained
2. 1 ripe avocado, mashed
3. 2 tablespoons coconut flour
4. 2 tablespoons chopped fresh chives
5. 1 teaspoon lemon juice
6. Coconut oil for frying
7. Salt to taste

INSTRUCTIONS:

1. In a bowl, combine drained tuna, mashed avocado, coconut flour, chopped chives, lemon juice, and salt.
2. Form the mixture into small patties.
3. Heat coconut oil in a skillet over medium heat. Fry tuna cakes for 3-4 minutes per side until golden brown.

Nutrition per Serving:

❖ Calories: 220
❖ Protein: 30g
❖ Fat: 10g
❖ Carbohydrates: 6g

AIP Coconut Lime Mahi Mahi

INGREDIENTS:

1. 4 mahi mahi fillets
2. ¼ cup coconut milk
3. 2 tablespoons fresh lime juice
4. 1 tablespoon coconut aminos
5. 2 cloves garlic, minced
6. 1 teaspoon grated ginger
7. Salt to taste

INSTRUCTIONS:

1. In a bowl, whisk together coconut milk, lime juice, coconut aminos, minced garlic, grated ginger, and salt.
2. Marinate mahi mahi fillets in the mixture for 20-30 minutes.
3. Preheat grill to medium-high heat. Grill fish for 4-5 minutes per side until cooked through.

Nutrition per Serving:

❖ Calories: 280
❖ Protein: 30g
❖ Fat: 12g
❖ Carbohydrates: 4g

AIP Lemon Herb Scallops

INGREDIENTS:

1. 1 pound scallops
2. 3 tablespoons olive oil
3. Zest of 1 lemon
4. 2 tablespoons chopped fresh parsley
5. 2 tablespoons chopped fresh dill
6. Salt to taste

INSTRUCTIONS:

1. Pat scallops dry and season with salt.
2. In a bowl, mix olive oil, lemon zest, chopped parsley, and chopped dill.
3. Heat a skillet over medium-high heat. Sear scallops for 2-3 minutes per side until golden and cooked through. Drizzle with the herb mixture while cooking.

Nutrition per Serving:

❖ Calories: 250
❖ Protein: 30g
❖ Fat: 12g
❖ Carbohydrates: 2g

AIP Shrimp and Zucchini Noodles

INGREDIENTS:

1. 1 pound shrimp, peeled and deveined
2. 4 medium zucchinis, spiralized into noodles
3. 2 tablespoons coconut oil
4. 2 cloves garlic, minced
5. 1 teaspoon fresh thyme leaves
6. Salt to taste

INSTRUCTIONS:

1. Heat coconut oil in a skillet over medium heat. Add minced garlic and thyme, sauté until fragrant.
2. Add shrimp and cook until pink.
3. Add zucchini noodles and sauté for 2-3 minutes until noodles are tender.
4. Season with salt and serve.

Nutrition per Serving:

- ❖ Calories: 220
- ❖ Protein: 28g
- ❖ Fat: 10g
- ❖ Carbohydrates: 8g

Wholesome AIP Beef, Pork, and Lamb Entrees

AIP Beef Stir-Fry

INGREDIENTS:

1. 1 lb grass-fed beef, thinly sliced
2. 2 cups broccoli florets
3. 1 onion, sliced
4. 3 garlic cloves, minced
5. 2 tablespoons coconut aminos
6. 2 tablespoons coconut oil
7. Salt and pepper (omit pepper for AIP)

INSTRUCTIONS:

1. Heat coconut oil in a skillet over medium heat.
2. Add beef slices and cook until browned. Remove from the skillet.
3. In the same skillet, sauté garlic, onion, and broccoli until tender.
4. Add beef back to the skillet, pour in coconut aminos, and stir-fry until heated through.
5. Season with salt to taste and serve.

Nutrition per Serving:

❖ Calories: 280 | Protein: 25g | Carbohydrates: 10g | Fat: 15gFat: 15g

AIP Beef and Vegetable Soup

INGREDIENTS:

1. 1 lb grass-fed beef, cubed
2. 4 cups bone broth
3. 2 carrots, chopped
4. 2 celery stalks, chopped
5. 1 sweet potato, diced
6. 2 garlic cloves, minced
7. 1 teaspoon turmeric powder
8. 1 bay leaf
9. Salt to taste

INSTRUCTIONS:

1. In a pot, brown beef cubes over medium heat.
2. Add bone broth, vegetables, garlic, turmeric, and bay leaf.
3. Simmer for 45 minutes to an hour until beef is tender.
4. Season with salt and serve hot.

Nutrition per Serving:

❖ Calories: 320 | Protein: 28g | Carbohydrates: 20g | Fat: 14g

AIP Beef and Plantain Skillet

INGREDIENTS:

1. 1 lb ground beef
2. 2 ripe plantains, sliced
3. 1 onion, diced
4. 2 garlic cloves, minced
5. 1 teaspoon turmeric powder
6. 2 tablespoons coconut oil
7. Salt to taste

INSTRUCTIONS:

1. In a skillet, heat coconut oil over medium heat.
2. Add onions and garlic, sauté until fragrant.
3. Add ground beef and cook until browned.
4. Add plantains and turmeric, cook until plantains are soft.
5. Season with salt and serve.

Nutrition per Serving:

❖ Calories: 340 | Protein: 22g | Carbohydrates: 28g | Fat: 16g

AIP Pork Entrees

INGREDIENTS:

1. 2 lbs pork shoulder, cubed
2. 1 onion, sliced
3. 3 garlic cloves, minced
4. 1 teaspoon ginger, grated
5. 2 cups bone broth
6. 2 tablespoons apple cider vinegar
7. Salt to taste

INSTRUCTIONS:

1. Place pork, onion, garlic, ginger, bone broth, and apple cider vinegar in a slow cooker.
2. Cook on low for 6-8 hours until pork is tender.
3. Shred the pork and season with salt before serving.

Nutrition per Serving:

❖ Calories: 280 | Protein: 30g | Carbohydrates: 5g | Fat: 14g

AIP Pork and Cabbage Stir-Fry

INGREDIENTS:

1. 1 lb pork loin, thinly sliced
2. 4 cups cabbage, shredded
3. 1 carrot, julienned
4. 2 green onions, chopped
5. 2 tablespoons coconut aminos
6. 2 tablespoons coconut oil
7. Salt to taste

INSTRUCTIONS:

1. Heat coconut oil in a skillet over medium heat.
2. Add pork slices and cook until browned. Remove from skillet.
3. Sauté cabbage, carrot, and green onions until tender.
4. Add pork back to the skillet, pour in coconut aminos, and stir-fry until heated through.
5. Season with salt and serve.

Nutrition per Serving:

❖ Calories: 310 | Protein: 25g | Carbohydrates: 15g | Fat: 16g

AIP Pork and Spinach Soup

INGREDIENTS:

1. 1 lb ground pork
2. 6 cups spinach leaves
3. 1 onion, diced
4. 3 garlic cloves, minced
5. 1 teaspoon turmeric powder
6. 4 cups bone broth
7. Salt to taste

INSTRUCTIONS:

1. Brown ground pork in a pot over medium heat.
2. Add onions and garlic, cook until translucent.
3. Stir in turmeric, bone broth, and simmer for 15 minutes.
4. Add spinach and cook until wilted.
5. Season with salt and serve hot.

Nutrition per Serving:

❖ Calories: 290 | Protein: 24g | Carbohydrates: 8g | Fat: 18g

AIP Lamb and Sweet Potato Hash

INGREDIENTS:

1. 1 lb ground lamb
2. 2 sweet potatoes, diced
3. 1 onion, diced
4. 2 garlic cloves, minced
5. 2 tablespoons coconut oil
6. 1 teaspoon dried rosemary
7. Salt to taste

INSTRUCTIONS:

1. Heat coconut oil in a skillet over medium heat.
2. Add onions and garlic, sauté until fragrant.
3. Add ground lamb and cook until browned.
4. Add sweet potatoes and rosemary, cook until sweet potatoes are tender.
5. Season with salt and serve.

Nutrition per Serving:

❖ Calories: 330 | Protein: 22g | Carbohydrates: 25g | Fat: 16g

AIP Lamb and Zucchini Skewers

INGREDIENTS:

1. 1 lb lamb cubes
2. 2 zucchinis, sliced
3. 1 lemon, juiced
4. 2 tablespoons olive oil
5. 2 garlic cloves, minced
6. 1 teaspoon dried oregano
7. Salt to taste

INSTRUCTIONS:

1. In a bowl, combine olive oil, lemon juice, garlic, oregano, and salt.
2. Marinate lamb cubes in the mixture for 30 minutes.
3. Thread lamb and zucchini slices onto skewers.
4. Grill or broil until lamb is cooked to desired doneness.
5. Serve hot.

Nutrition per Serving:

❖ Calories: 300 | Protein: 24g | Carbohydrates: 10g | Fat: 18g

AIP Lamb and Cauliflower Rice Bowl

INGREDIENTS:

1. 1 lb lamb chops
2. 4 cups cauliflower rice
3. 1 bell pepper, diced
4. 1 onion, sliced
5. 2 tablespoons coconut oil
6. 1 teaspoon turmeric powder
7. Salt to taste

INSTRUCTIONS:

1. Heat coconut oil in a skillet over medium heat.
2. Sear lamb chops until cooked to desired doneness. Remove and set aside.
3. Sauté onions, bell pepper, and cauliflower rice until tender.
4. Stir in turmeric and season with salt.
5. Serve the lamb chops over the cauliflower rice mixture.

Nutrition per Serving:

❖ Calories: 340 | Protein: 26g | Carbohydrates: 15g | Fat: 20g

AIP Lamb and Carrot Curry

INGREDIENTS:

1. 1 lb lamb stew meat
2. 4 carrots, sliced
3. 1 onion, diced
4. 3 garlic cloves, minced
5. 1-inch fresh ginger, grated
6. 2 cups coconut milk
7. 2 tablespoons curry powder (AIP-compliant)
8. 2 tablespoons coconut oil
9. Salt to taste

INSTRUCTIONS:

1. In a pot, heat coconut oil over medium heat.
2. Sauté onions, garlic, and ginger until fragrant.
3. Add lamb and brown on all sides.
4. Stir in curry powder, carrots, and coconut milk.
5. Simmer for 1-1.5 hours until lamb is tender.
6. Season with salt and serve with cauliflower rice.

Nutrition per Serving:

❖ Calories: 370 | Protein: 24g | Carbohydrates: 18g | Fat: 24g

Chapter 6

DELECTABLE SIDES AND SNACKS

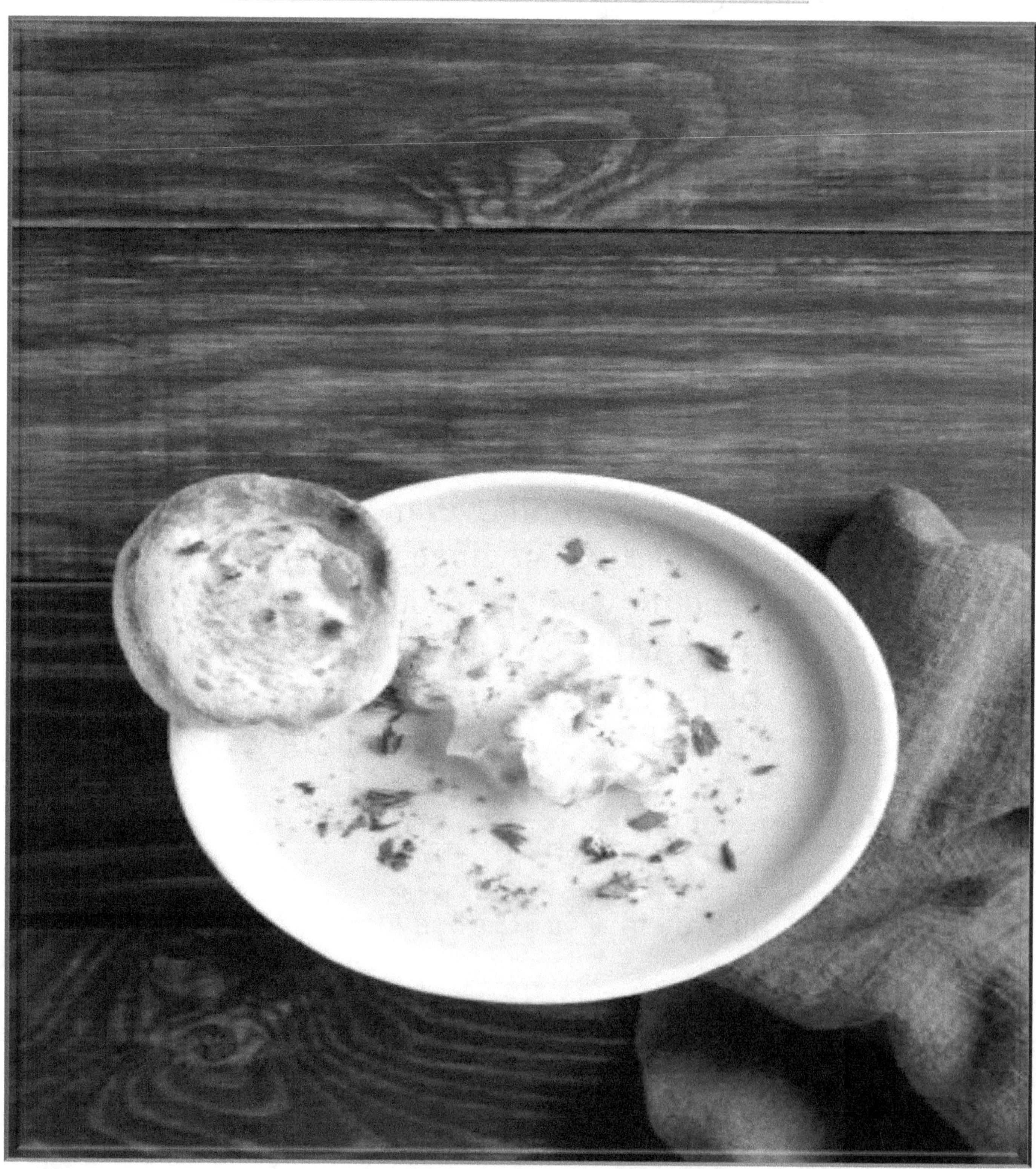

Roasted Garlic Cauliflower Mash

INGREDIENTS:

1. 1 head cauliflower, chopped
2. 2 cloves garlic, minced
3. 2 tbsp coconut oil
4. Salt to taste

INSTRUCTIONS:

1. Preheat oven to 400°F (200°C).
2. Toss cauliflower and garlic with coconut oil, sprinkle with salt.
3. Roast for 25-30 minutes until tender.
4. Mash roasted cauliflower until smooth.

Nutrition per Serving:

❖ Calories: 80
❖ Carbohydrates: 6g
❖ Fat: 6g
❖ Protein: 3g

Baked Sweet Potato Fries

INGREDIENTS:

1. 2 medium sweet potatoes, cut into fries
2. 2 tbsp avocado oil
3. Sea salt to taste

INSTRUCTIONS:

1. Preheat oven to 425°F (220°C).
2. Toss sweet potatoes with avocado oil and salt.
3. Bake for 20-25 minutes until crispy.

Nutrition per Serving:

❖ Calories: 120
❖ Carbohydrates: 26g
❖ Fat: 3g
❖ Protein: 2g

Garlic Herb Roasted Carrots

INGREDIENTS:

1. 1 lb carrots, peeled and sliced
2. 2 tbsp olive oil
3. 2 cloves garlic, minced
4. Fresh herbs (rosemary/thyme)
5. Salt and pepper to taste

INSTRUCTIONS:

1. Preheat oven to 400°F (200°C).
2. Toss carrots, garlic, herbs, olive oil, salt, and pepper.
3. Roast for 20-25 minutes until tender.

Nutrition per Serving:

❖ Calories: 80
❖ Carbohydrates: 12g
❖ Fat: 4g
❖ Protein: 1g

Zucchini Noodles with Pesto

INGREDIENTS:

1. 3 medium zucchinis, spiralized
2. ¼ cup AIP-friendly pesto
3. Salt and pepper to taste

INSTRUCTIONS:

1. Sauté zucchini noodles in a pan until tender.
2. Toss with AIP pesto, salt, and pepper.

Nutrition per Serving:

- ❖ Calories: 50
- ❖ Carbohydrates: 5g
- ❖ Fat: 3g
- ❖ Protein: 2g

Ginger-Glazed Bok Choy

INGREDIENTS:

1. 4 baby bok choy, halved
2. 2 tbsp coconut aminos
3. 1 tsp grated ginger
4. 1 tbsp coconut oil

INSTRUCTIONS:

1. Heat coconut oil in a pan, add bok choy, ginger, and coconut aminos.
2. Sauté for 5-7 minutes until tender.

Nutrition per Serving:

❖ Calories: 30
❖ Carbohydrates: 4g
❖ Fat: 2g
❖ Protein: 2g

Turmeric-Ginger Mashed Sweet Potatoes

INGREDIENTS:

1. 2 medium sweet potatoes, boiled
2. 1 tsp turmeric powder
3. 1 tsp grated ginger
4. Salt to taste

INSTRUCTIONS:

1. Mash boiled sweet potatoes with turmeric, ginger, and salt.

Nutrition per Serving:

- ❖ Calories: 120
- ❖ Carbohydrates: 28g
- ❖ Fat: 0g
- ❖ Protein: 2g

Roasted Brussels Sprouts with Bacon

INGREDIENTS:

2. 1 lb Brussels sprouts, halved
3. 4 slices AIP-compliant bacon, chopped
4. 2 tbsp olive oil
5. Salt and pepper to taste

INSTRUCTIONS:

1. Toss Brussels sprouts and bacon with olive oil, salt, and pepper.
2. Roast for 25-30 minutes until crispy.

Nutrition per Serving:

❖ Calories: 100
❖ Carbohydrates: 8g
❖ Fat: 7g
❖ Protein: 5g

Mashed Butternut Squash

INGREDIENTS:

1. 1 medium butternut squash, peeled and cubed
2. 2 tbsp coconut oil
3. Cinnamon (optional)
4. Salt to taste

INSTRUCTIONS:

1. Boil or steam squash until tender.
2. Mash with coconut oil, cinnamon (if using), and salt.

Nutrition per Serving:

❖ Calories: 80
❖ Carbohydrates: 22g
❖ Fat: 4g
❖ Protein: 1g

Ginger-Garlic Green Beans

INGREDIENTS:

1. 1 lb green beans, trimmed
2. 2 cloves garlic, minced
3. 1 tsp grated ginger
4. 1 tbsp coconut aminos
5. 1 tbsp olive oil

INSTRUCTIONS:

1. Heat olive oil in a pan, add garlic, ginger, and green beans.
2. Sauté for 8-10 minutes until tender.
3. Add coconut aminos, toss, and serve.

Nutrition per Serving:

❖ Calories: 60
❖ Carbohydrates: 8g
❖ Fat: 3g
❖ Protein: 2g

Crispy Turnip Fries

INGREDIENTS:

1. 2 large turnips, cut into fries
2. 2 tbsp coconut oil
3. Sea salt to taste

INSTRUCTIONS:

1. Toss turnip fries with coconut oil and salt.
2. Bake at 425°F (220°C) for 25-30 minutes until crispy.

Nutrition per Serving:

- ❖ Calories: 50
- ❖ Carbohydrates: 10g
- ❖ Fat: 3g
- ❖ Protein: 1g

Berry Coconut Breakfast Bowl

INGREDIENTS:

9. 1 cup mixed berries (blueberries, raspberries, strawberries)
10. 1/2 cup shredded coconut
11. 1 tablespoon chia seeds
12. Coconut milk (as needed for desired consistency)

INSTRUCTIONS:

8. Blend mixed berries and coconut milk until smooth.
9. Pour the berry mixture into a bowl.
10. Top with shredded coconut and chia seeds.

Nutrition per Serving:

- ❖ Calories: 220
- ❖ Protein: 3g
- ❖ Carbohydrates: 20g
- ❖ Fat: 15g

Baked Sweet Potato Chips

INGREDIENTS:

1. 2 medium sweet potatoes
2. 2 tablespoons coconut oil, melted
3. Sea salt to taste

INSTRUCTIONS:

1. Preheat oven to 225°F (110°C).
2. Thinly slice sweet potatoes using a mandoline slicer or a sharp knife.
3. Toss the slices in melted coconut oil and sprinkle with sea salt.
4. Place the slices on a baking sheet lined with parchment paper, ensuring they don't overlap.
5. Bake for 1.5 to 2 hours until crispy, flipping the slices halfway through.
6. Let them cool to crisp up further before enjoying.

Nutrition per Serving:

❖ Calories: 120
❖ Fat: 7g
❖ Carbohydrates: 14g
❖ Fiber: 2.5g
❖ Protein: 1g

Crispy Kale Chips

INGREDIENTS:

1. 1 bunch kale, stems removed and torn into bite-sized pieces
2. 1 tablespoon olive oil
3. Sea salt or AIP-friendly seasoning blend

INSTRUCTIONS:

1. Preheat oven to 275°F (135°C).
2. Toss kale pieces with olive oil in a large bowl, ensuring they're evenly coated.
3. Spread the kale on a baking sheet lined with parchment paper.
4. Sprinkle with sea salt or AIP-friendly seasoning.
5. Bake for 20-25 minutes until crispy, but not burnt.
6. Let them cool before serving.

Nutrition per Serving:

❖ Calories: 50
❖ Fat: 3g
❖ Carbohydrates: 5g
❖ Fiber: 1.5g
❖ Protein: 1.5g

Plantain Chips

INGREDIENTS:

1. 2 green plantains
2. 3 tablespoons coconut oil
3. Sea salt to taste

INSTRUCTIONS:

1. Preheat oven to 350°F (175°C).
2. Peel plantains and thinly slice using a mandoline slicer or knife.
3. Toss slices in melted coconut oil and sprinkle with sea salt.
4. Place slices on a baking sheet lined with parchment paper.
5. Bake for 20-25 minutes, flipping halfway through, until golden brown.
6. Let them cool and crisp up before serving.

Nutrition per Serving:

- Calories: 150
- Fat: 9g
- Carbohydrates: 18g
- Fiber: 1.5g
- Protein: 1g

Crispy Apple Chips

INGREDIENTS:

1. 2 apples, cored and thinly sliced
2. 1 tablespoon lemon juice
3. Cinnamon (optional)

INSTRUCTIONS:

1. Preheat oven to 200°F (95°C).
2. Toss apple slices in lemon juice to prevent browning.
3. Place slices on a baking sheet lined with parchment paper.
4. Sprinkle with cinnamon if desired.
5. Bake for 1.5 to 2 hours until crispy, flipping slices halfway through.
6. Let them cool completely before serving.

Nutrition per Serving:

❖ Calories: 60
❖ Fat: 0.5g
❖ Carbohydrates: 16g
❖ Fiber: 3g
❖ Protein: 0.5g

Roasted Spiced Nuts

INGREDIENTS:

1. 2 cups mixed AIP-friendly nuts (almonds, cashews, macadamias)
2. 1 tablespoon melted coconut oil
3. AIP-friendly spices (e.g., cinnamon, ginger, or turmeric)

INSTRUCTIONS:

1. Preheat oven to 300°F (150°C).
2. Toss nuts in melted coconut oil and sprinkle with chosen spices.
3. Spread nuts on a baking sheet lined with parchment paper.
4. Roast for 15-20 minutes, stirring occasionally, until fragrant and golden.
5. Let them cool before enjoying..

Nutrition per Serving:

❖ Calories: 180
❖ Fat: 16g
❖ Carbohydrates: 7g
❖ Fiber: 3g
❖ Protein: 5g

Creamy Avocado Dip

INGREDIENTS:

1. 2 ripe avocados
2. 1 tablespoon fresh lemon juice
3. 2 tablespoons chopped fresh cilantro
4. 1 clove garlic, minced
5. Salt to taste

INSTRUCTIONS:

1. Cut avocados in half, remove pits, and scoop the flesh into a bowl.
2. Mash the avocados with a fork until smooth.
3. Add lemon juice, chopped cilantro, minced garlic, and salt. Mix until well combined.
4. Adjust seasoning to taste.
5. Serve immediately or refrigerate for later use.

Nutrition per Serving:

- ❖ Calories: 120
- ❖ Total Fat: 11g
- ❖ Carbohydrates: 7g
- ❖ Fiber: 5g
- ❖ Protein: 2g

Garlic Herb Dressing

INGREDIENTS:

1. ½ cup extra virgin olive oil
2. 2 tablespoons apple cider vinegar
3. 1 tablespoon chopped fresh parsley
4. 1 teaspoon minced garlic
5. Salt and pepper to taste

INSTRUCTIONS:

1. In a jar, combine olive oil, apple cider vinegar, chopped parsley, minced garlic, salt, and pepper.
2. Secure the lid and shake vigorously until well emulsified.
3. Adjust salt and pepper to taste.
4. Drizzle over salads or use as a marinade.

Nutrition per Serving:

- Calories: 80
- Total Fat: 9g
- Carbohydrates: 0g
- Fiber: 0g
- Protein: 0g

Cilantro Lime Avocado Sauce

INGREDIENTS:

1. 1 ripe avocado
2. Juice of 2 limes
3. Handful of fresh cilantro leaves
4. 1 tablespoon extra virgin olive oil
5. Salt to taste

INSTRUCTIONS:

1. Blend avocado, lime juice, cilantro, and olive oil in a food processor until smooth.
2. Add salt to taste and blend again until well combined.
3. Adjust lime juice or salt as needed.
4. Use as a sauce for grilled meats or as a dip for vegetables.

Nutrition per Serving:

❖ Calories: 25
❖ Total Fat: 2g
❖ Carbohydrates: 1g
❖ Fiber: 1g
❖ Protein: 0g

Beetroot Hummus

INGREDIENTS:

1. 1 medium-sized beetroot, roasted and peeled
2. 1 can (15 oz) cooked and drained white sweet potatoes
3. 2 tablespoons tahini
4. Juice of 1 lemon
5. 1 clove garlic, minced
6. Salt to taste

INSTRUCTIONS:

1. In a food processor, blend roasted beetroot, cooked sweet potatoes, tahini, lemon juice, minced garlic, and salt until smooth.
2. Adjust seasoning to taste and add more lemon juice if desired.
3. Serve as a dip with vegetable sticks or use as a spread.

Nutrition per Serving:

* Calories: 70
* Total Fat: 2g
* Carbohydrates: 12g
* Fiber: 2g
* Protein: 1g

Mango Salsa

INGREDIENTS:

1. 1 ripe mango, diced
2. 1/2 red onion, finely chopped
3. 1 red bell pepper, diced
4. Juice of 1 lime
5. Handful of fresh cilantro, chopped
6. Salt to taste

INSTRUCTIONS:

1. In a bowl, combine diced mango, chopped red onion, diced red bell pepper, lime juice, and chopped cilantro.
2. Season with salt to taste and mix well.
3. Refrigerate for at least 30 minutes before serving to allow flavors to meld.
4. Serve with grilled chicken or fish.

Nutrition per Serving:

❖ Calories: 35
❖ Total Fat: 0g
❖ Carbohydrates: 9g
❖ Fiber: 1g
❖ Protein: 0g

Chapter 7

Indulgent AIP Desserts

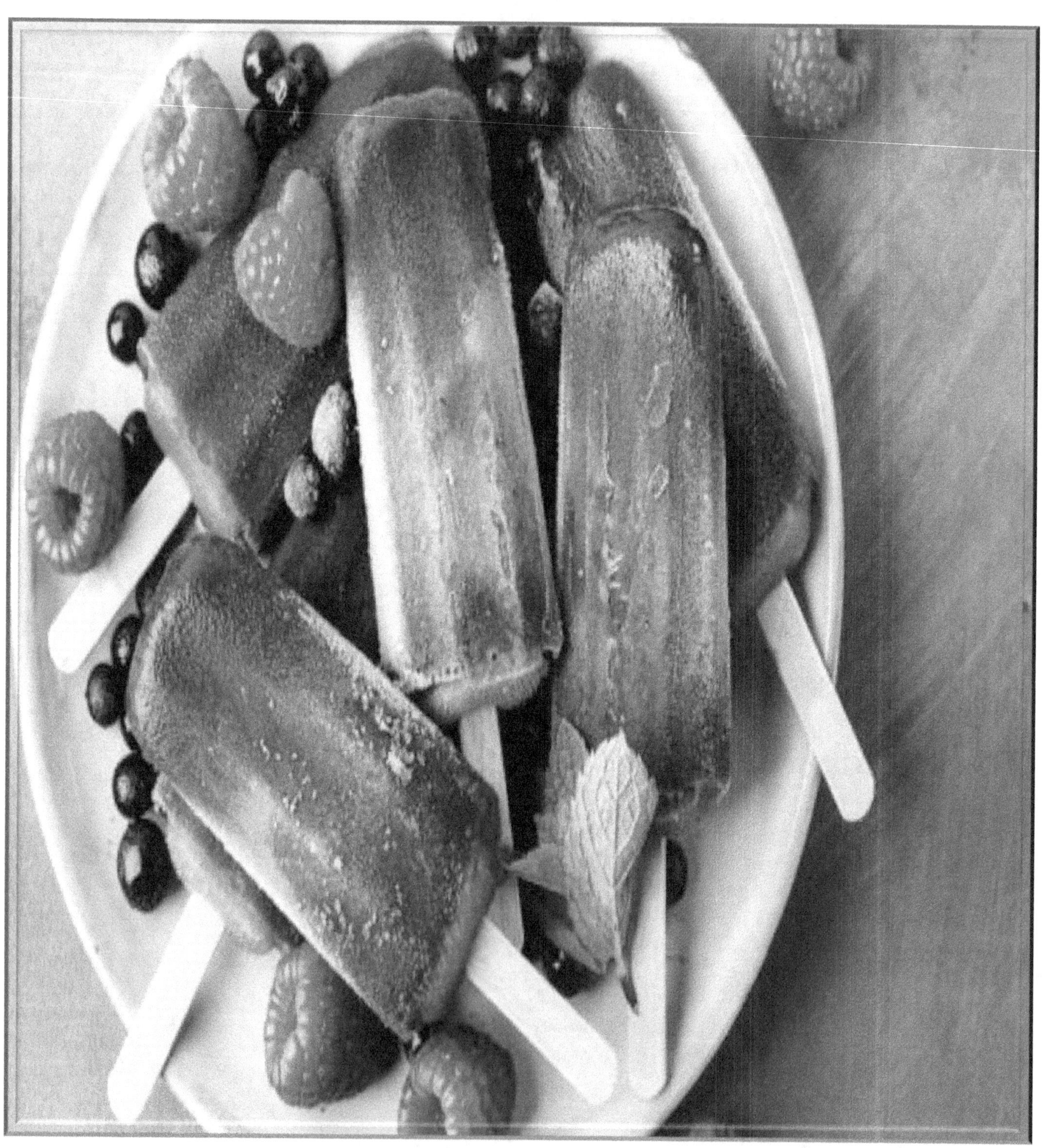

AIP Blueberry Coconut Popsicles

INGREDIENTS:

1. 1 cup fresh blueberries
2. 1 can (13.5 oz) coconut milk
3. 2 tablespoons raw honey
4. 1 teaspoon vanilla extract (AIP-compliant)

INSTRUCTIONS:

1. Blend blueberries, coconut milk, honey, and vanilla extract until smooth.
2. Pour the mixture into popsicle molds.
3. Freeze for at least 4 hours or until set.
4. Serve and enjoy!

Nutrition per Serving:

- ❖ Calories: 120
- ❖ Carbohydrates: 12g
- ❖ Fat: 8g
- ❖ Protein: 1g

AIP Carrot Cake Bites

INGREDIENTS:

1. 1 cup shredded carrots
2. 1 cup unsweetened shredded coconut
3. ½ cup medjool dates (pitted)
4. ½ cup unsweetened applesauce
5. 1 teaspoon ground cinnamon
6. ¼ teaspoon ground ginger
7. Pinch of sea salt

INSTRUCTIONS:

1. Blend carrots, shredded coconut, dates, applesauce, cinnamon, ginger, and salt until a dough forms.
2. Roll the mixture into bite-sized balls.
3. Place in the refrigerator for 30 minutes to set.
4. Serve chilled.

Nutrition per Serving:

❖ Calories: 110
❖ Carbohydrates: 18g
❖ Fat: 4g
❖ Protein: 1g

AIP Strawberry Banana "Nice" Cream

INGREDIENTS:

1. 2 ripe bananas (sliced and frozen)
2. 1 cup frozen strawberries
3. ¼ cup coconut cream
4. 1 tablespoon raw honey (optional)

INSTRUCTIONS:

1. Blend frozen bananas, strawberries, coconut cream, and honey until smooth and creamy.
2. Serve immediately as soft-serve "nice" cream or freeze for a firmer texture.

Nutrition per Serving:

❖ Calories: 120
❖ Carbohydrates: 28g
❖ Fat: 3g
❖ Protein: 1g

AIP Lemon Coconut Bliss Balls

INGREDIENTS:

1. 1 cup unsweetened shredded coconut
2. Zest of 1 lemon
3. 2 tablespoons coconut butter
4. 2 tablespoons raw honey
5. 1 tablespoon lemon juice

INSTRUCTIONS:

1. Combine shredded coconut, lemon zest, coconut butter, honey, and lemon juice in a food processor. Pulse until well combined.
2. Roll the mixture into small balls.
3. Refrigerate for 30 minutes before serving.

Nutrition per Serving:

- ❖ Calories: 90
- ❖ Carbohydrates: 6g
- ❖ Fat: 7g
- ❖ Protein: 1g

AIP Cinnamon Baked Apples

INGREDIENTS:

1. 2 apples (cored and halved)
2. 2 tablespoons coconut oil (melted)
3. 1 teaspoon ground cinnamon
4. 2 tablespoons unsweetened shredded coconut (optional)

INSTRUCTIONS:

1. Preheat oven to 350°F (175°C).
2. Place apple halves on a baking sheet.
3. Drizzle melted coconut oil over apples, sprinkle with cinnamon, and add shredded coconut if desired.
4. Bake for 25-30 minutes or until apples are tender.
5. Serve warm.

Nutrition per Serving:

❖ Calories: 90
❖ Carbohydrates: 12g
❖ Fat: 5g
❖ Protein: 0.5g

Baked Cinnamon Apples

INGREDIENTS:

1. 4 medium-sized apples, cored and sliced
2. 1 tablespoon melted coconut oil
3. 1 teaspoon cinnamon
4. 1 tablespoon maple syrup (optional)
5. Juice of half a lemon

INSTRUCTIONS:

1. Preheat the oven to 350°F (175°C).
2. In a bowl, toss the apple slices with melted coconut oil, cinnamon, and maple syrup (if using).
3. Squeeze lemon juice over the apples and mix gently.
4. Place the coated apple slices in a baking dish.
5. Bake for 20-25 minutes until the apples are tender.
6. Serve warm as a delightful dessert or snack.

Nutrition per Serving:

- ❖ Calories: 100
- ❖ Total Fat: 3g
- ❖ Total Carbohydrates: 22g
- ❖ Fiber: 5g
- ❖ Sugars: 16g
- ❖ Protein: 0.5g

Berry Coconut Popsicles

INGREDIENTS:

1. 1 cup mixed berries (such as strawberries, blueberries, raspberries)
2. 1 can (13.5 oz) coconut milk
3. 1 tablespoon raw honey (optional)

INSTRUCTIONS:

1. Blend the mixed berries and coconut milk until smooth.
2. Sweeten with raw honey if desired.
3. Pour the mixture into popsicle molds.
4. Freeze for at least 4-6 hours until solid.
5. Run the molds under warm water to release the popsicles before serving.

Nutrition per Serving:

❖ Calories: 90
❖ Total Fat: 8g
❖ Total Carbohydrates: 5g
❖ Fiber: 1.5g
❖ Sugars: 3g
❖ Protein: 1g

Pineapple Coconut Chia Pudding

INGREDIENTS:

1. 1 cup diced pineapple
2. 1 can (13.5 oz) coconut milk
3. 3 tablespoons chia seeds
4. 1 tablespoon maple syrup (optional)

INSTRUCTIONS:

1. Blend the diced pineapple and coconut milk until smooth.
2. Pour the mixture into a bowl and stir in the chia seeds.
3. Sweeten with maple syrup if desired.
4. Refrigerate for at least 2-3 hours or overnight until the chia seeds expand and create a pudding-like consistency.
5. Serve chilled with a sprinkle of shredded coconut on top.

Nutrition per Serving:

❖ Calories: 220
❖ Total Fat: 18g
❖ Total Carbohydrates: 15g
❖ Fiber: 6g
❖ Sugars: 8g
❖ Protein: 3g

Mango Banana "Nice Cream"

INGREDIENTS:

1. 2 ripe bananas, sliced and frozen
2. 1 ripe mango, peeled and cubed
3. 1 tablespoon coconut milk (if needed for blending)

INSTRUCTIONS:

1. Place the frozen banana slices and mango cubes in a blender or food processor.
2. Blend until smooth, adding coconut milk if needed for creaminess.
3. Transfer the mixture into a bowl.
4. Serve immediately for a creamy, ice cream-like treat.

Nutrition per Serving:

- ❖ Calories: 150
- ❖ Total Fat: 0.5g
- ❖ Total Carbohydrates: 38g
- ❖ Fiber: 5g
- ❖ Sugars: 24g
- ❖ Protein: 2g

Baked Pears with Honey and Cinnamon

INGREDIENTS:

1. 4 ripe pears, halved and cored
2. 2 tablespoons raw honey
3. 1 teaspoon cinnamon

INSTRUCTIONS:

1. Preheat the oven to 375°F (190°C).
2. Place the pear halves, cut side up, on a baking sheet lined with parchment paper.
3. Drizzle each pear half with raw honey and sprinkle with cinnamon.
4. Bake for 30-35 minutes until the pears are tender and caramelized.
5. Serve warm as a comforting dessert..

Nutrition per Serving:

- ❖ Calories: 120
- ❖ Total Fat: 0.5g
- ❖ Total Carbohydrates: 32g
- ❖ Fiber: 6g
- ❖ Sugars: 23g
- ❖ Protein: 1g

AIP Blueberry Muffins

INGREDIENTS:

1. 2 cups tiger nut flour
2. 1/2 cup coconut flour
3. 1/4 cup maple syrup
4. 1/3 cup coconut oil (melted)
5. 1/2 cup applesauce
6. 1 tsp baking soda
7. 1/2 tsp cinnamon
8. 1 cup fresh blueberries

INSTRUCTIONS:

1. Preheat the oven to 350°F (175°C). Line a muffin tin with paper liners.
2. In a mixing bowl, combine tiger nut flour, coconut flour, baking soda, and cinnamon.
3. Stir in the melted coconut oil, maple syrup, and applesauce until well combined.
4. Gently fold in the fresh blueberries.
5. Divide the batter evenly among the muffin cups.
6. Bake for 25-30 minutes or until a toothpick inserted into the center comes out clean.
7. Allow muffins to cool before serving.

Nutrition per Serving:

- ❖ Calories: 180
- ❖ Protein: 3g
- ❖ Carbohydrates: 20g
- ❖ Fat: 10g
- ❖ Fiber: 5g

AIP Banana Bread

INGREDIENTS:

1. 3 ripe bananas
2. 3/4 cup coconut flour
3. 1/4 cup coconut oil (melted)
4. 3 tbsp maple syrup
5. 1 tsp baking soda
6. 1 tsp cinnamon
7. Pinch of salt

INSTRUCTIONS:

1. Preheat oven to 350°F (175°C). Grease a loaf pan.
2. In a mixing bowl, mash the ripe bananas.
3. Add melted coconut oil, maple syrup, and mix well.
4. Stir in coconut flour, baking soda, cinnamon, and salt until combined.
5. Pour the batter into the prepared loaf pan.
6. Bake for 40-45 minutes or until a toothpick inserted in the center comes out clean.
7. Allow the banana bread to cool completely before slicing.

Nutrition per Serving:

❖ Calories: 160
❖ Protein: 2g
❖ Carbohydrates: 20g
❖ Fat: 8g
❖ Fiber: 6g

AIP Carrot Cake Cupcakes

INGREDIENTS:

1. 2 cups shredded carrots
2. 1/2 cup coconut flour
3. 1/4 cup coconut oil (melted)
4. 1/3 cup maple syrup
5. 3 eggs (or flax eggs for AIP-friendly option)
6. 1 tsp baking soda
7. 1 tsp cinnamon
8. 1/4 tsp ground ginger

INSTRUCTIONS:

1. Preheat oven to 350°F (175°C). Line a cupcake tin with paper liners.
2. In a bowl, mix shredded carrots, coconut flour, baking soda, cinnamon, and ground ginger.
3. Add melted coconut oil, maple syrup, and eggs; mix until well combined.
4. Divide the batter evenly into the cupcake liners.
5. Bake for 20-25 minutes or until a toothpick comes out clean.
6. Allow cupcakes to cool before frosting (optional).

Nutrition per Serving:

❖ Calories: 150
❖ Protein: 3g
❖ Carbohydrates: 15g
❖ Fat: 8g
❖ Fiber: 5g

AIP Pumpkin Spice Cookies

INGREDIENTS:

1. 1 cup pumpkin puree
2. 1/2 cup coconut flour
3. 1/4 cup coconut oil (melted)
4. 1/4 cup maple syrup
5. 1 tsp cinnamon
6. 1/2 tsp ground ginger
7. 1/4 tsp ground cloves
8. 1/4 tsp baking soda
9. Pinch of salt

INSTRUCTIONS:

1. Preheat oven to 350°F (175°C). Line a baking sheet with parchment paper.
2. In a bowl, mix pumpkin puree, melted coconut oil, and maple syrup.
3. Add coconut flour, cinnamon, ginger, cloves, baking soda, and salt; mix until a dough forms.
4. Scoop out tablespoon-sized portions and place them on the baking sheet.
5. Flatten each cookie slightly with a fork.
6. Bake for 18-20 minutes or until lightly golden.
7. Let the cookies cool completely before enjoying.

Nutrition per Serving:

❖ Calories: 110
❖ Protein: 2g
❖ Carbohydrates: 10g
❖ Fat: 7g
❖ Fiber: 4g

AIP Lemon Coconut Bars

INGREDIENTS:

1. 1 cup coconut flour
2. 1/2 cup coconut oil (melted)
3. 1/4 cup maple syrup
4. Zest and juice of 2 lemons
5. 1/2 cup shredded coconut (unsweetened)
6. Pinch of salt

INSTRUCTIONS:

1. Preheat oven to 350°F (175°C). Grease a square baking dish.
2. In a bowl, combine coconut flour, melted coconut oil, maple syrup, lemon zest, lemon juice, shredded coconut, and a pinch of salt. Mix until a crumbly dough forms.
3. Press the dough evenly into the baking dish.
4. Bake for 20-25 minutes or until the edges turn golden brown.
5. Let it cool completely before cutting into bars.

Nutrition per Serving:

❖ Calories: 120

❖ Protein: 2g

❖ Carbohydrates: 10g

❖ Fat: 8g

❖ Fiber: 5g

Tips for Staying AIP Compliant at Social Gatherings

It may be both enjoyable and difficult to follow the Autoimmune Paleo Protocol (AIP) and socialize at the same time. The following crucial advice can help you stay compliant while having fun at social events:

Be Informed Ahead of Time: Let guests or hosts know about your dietary needs and gently explain that you follow the AIP. Make sure there is something you can eat by offering to bring food that complies with your dietary requirements.

Plan Ahead: Eat a filling AIP-compliant meal before going to avoid the need to eat anything non-compliant out of desperation.

Make Smart Decisions: Consider all of your selections and concentrate on the whole meals that are being served at the event. For simpler, more AIP-compliant meals, go for grilled meats, fresh veggies, or fruit platters.

Bring your snacks, or BYOS for short-term weight loss. Fruit, vegetable sticks, or handmade AIP goodies are portable and may help you stay satiated if there aren't many alternatives.

Politely Reject Non-Compliant Foods: Acknowledge your dietary limits and politely dismiss any items that don't follow the AIP, without feeling forced to provide a detailed explanation.

Enjoy the Company: Reorient the conversation away from the meal and toward mingling and having fun. Celebrate the event for the relationships and learning opportunities it provides, which go beyond the food.

To ensure that you follow the rules and have fun at the social event, it's important to prepare, communicate, and have a good attitude while navigating social settings on AIP.

How to Dine Out While Following AIP

It takes some preparation and discussion to follow the Autoimmune Paleo Protocol (AIP) while dining out. Here's how to manage eating out while adhering to the AIP:

Investigate Now: Look for eateries that provide options for AIP adaptations on their menus. Choose restaurants that respect dietary restrictions and have an emphasis on serving healthy meals.

Make a Reservation or Look Up Menus Online: Give the restaurant a call ahead of time to discuss your dietary requirements. Find out whether they will alter recipes or take AIP limits into account. AIP-friendly choices may also be marked on online menus.

Communicate Clearly: Let the server know about any dietary limitations you may have before you arrive. Kindly inquire whether they can make meals without certain items, such as dairy, wheat, or specific spices that are utilized in recipes that are not compliant.

Simplify Orders: Go for simple foods like salads with dressings that are permitted by the AIP, steaming veggies, or grilled meats. It's usually possible to customize orders by leaving out elements that don't comply.

Bring Your Own Sauce/Dressing (BYOS): If the restaurant's selections don't follow the protocol, think about bringing your condiments or dressings that have been authorized by the AIP to go with your meal.

Remain Mindful and Adaptable: Remain open to changing your mind in response to new information. Give more importance to the company and the eating experience than just the food.

Eating out while sticking to the AIP may be easy and fun if you talk to the restaurant staff, look into your alternatives, and are flexible.

Handling Challenges and Staying Motivated

There are obstacles to navigating the Autoimmune Paleo Protocol (AIP), but persistence in motivation are essential for success:

Become Informed: Recognize the theory behind AIP and its possible advantages in the treatment of autoimmune diseases. Acquiring knowledge strengthens and validates your dedication.

Accept Progress Rather Than Perfection: Acknowledge that obstacles can arise. Celebrate your tiny triumphs and the good adjustments you're making rather than dwelling on your mistakes.

Find Support: After AIP, get in touch with local communities, internet discussion boards, or support groups. Exchanging insights and advice may increase drive and provide priceless support.

Plan and Prepare: To reduce impulsive decisions or feeling unprepared, give meal planning, storing AIP-friendly foods, and snack preparation a top priority.

Emphasis on Wellness: Instead of concentrating on dietary limitations, draw attention to the general increase in well-being. Keep track of the other ways that AIP improves your health beyond symptom relief.

Exercise Self-Compassion: Treat yourself with kindness. Recognize the difficulties, but in your approach to adhering to AIP, be kind and supportive.

Maintaining motivation while following the AIP requires endurance, patience, and keeping the bigger picture of better health and well-being in mind. Honor your efforts and accomplishments, and never forget that every step you take ahead is evidence of your hard work.

Chapter 9

Importance of Stress Management in AIP

Effective stress management is essential to the Autoimmune Paleo Protocol (AIP)'s effectiveness for those with autoimmune diseases. The immune system may be greatly impacted by stress, which can worsen symptoms by inducing inflammatory reactions. The following explains why stress management in the AIP environment is essential:

Effect on Inflammation: One of the main causes of autoimmune illnesses is chronic stress, which raises the body's levels of inflammation. Techniques for managing stress may lessen this inflammatory reaction.

The relationship between stress and gut health: Stress increases gut permeability, which may lead to a leaky gut, a condition associated with autoimmune diseases. People who practice stress management promote gut health and facilitate the healing process which is essential to AIP.

Immune Function: Stress impairs immunity, increasing the risk of autoimmune responses or flare-ups. Putting stress management techniques into practice boosts the immune system.

General Health: AIP emphasizes general health. In addition to lowering stress, stress-reduction methods like deep breathing, yoga, meditation, or mindfulness also improve mental and emotional health, which is why they are a good addition to the AIP diet.

When implementing the Autoimmune Paleo Protocol, prioritizing stress management in addition to dietary adjustments guarantees a more thorough approach to controlling autoimmune disorders and aids in the body's healing process.

Exercise and AIP: Finding Balance

Exercise is an important part of an all-encompassing strategy while implementing the Autoimmune Paleo Protocol (AIP). For those who are managing autoimmune disorders, finding the ideal balance in activity is essential:

Low-Impact Exercises: Especially in the early stages of AIP, choose low-impact activities like yoga, strolling, swimming, or light cycling. Without overstretching the body, these exercises support circulation and preserve mobility.

Stress Management: One useful tactic for reducing stress is exercise. However strenuous exercise could raise stress levels, which might affect autoimmune diseases. It's crucial to strike a balance between stress-relieving hobbies and intense exercise.

Listen to Your Body: Observe how various types of exercise affect your body's response. Adapt the style, length, and intensity of your workout to your level of discomfort. When necessary, take a nap, and refrain from going beyond your limit.

Gradual Progression: Think about progressively adding mild exercise or strength training as your symptoms get better and your energy levels settle while on AIP. Begin with brief workouts and gradually ramp up the intensity.

General Well-Being: Exercise should support the AIP's all-encompassing methodology. Along with your workout regimen, pay attention to maintaining overall well-being, which includes stress management, enough sleep, and a balanced diet.

People may strike a balance that enhances physical well-being without aggravating autoimmune symptoms by seeing exercise as a supporting component of AIP, which will favorably impact their health journey.

Sleep and Its Impact on Autoimmune Health

Sleep has a major impact on the immune system's performance and general health, which is important for autoimmune wellness:

Immune Function: Having a strong immune system depends on getting enough sleep. Getting enough sleep is important for immune cell formation and activity, which helps the body fight off infections and control immunological responses. These functions are critical for the management of autoimmune diseases.

Control of Inflammation: Lack of sleep or irregular sleep schedules may cause the body to become more inflammatory. A prevalent characteristic of autoimmune disorders is increased inflammation. Getting enough sleep might help control inflammatory pathways, which may lessen the symptoms of autoimmune diseases.

Gut Health: Sleep has an impact on gut health, which is crucial for autoimmune diseases. Sleep disturbances have the potential to affect the gut flora and exacerbate autoimmune diseases linked to the gut. Sufficient sleep promotes a healthy gut environment.

Stress Management: There is a connection between stress and sleep. Sleep deprivation raises stress hormone levels, which might affect immune system performance and perhaps lead to flare-ups of autoimmune disease. Good sleep promotes general health by lowering stress.

Recuperation and Healing: The body goes through processes of regeneration and repair when you sleep. This includes hormone modulation, tissue healing, and cellular renewal—all crucial components in the treatment of autoimmune diseases and the enhancement of general health.

Making enough sleep a priority is essential for maintaining autoimmune health while adhering to the Autoimmune Paleo Protocol (AIP). Immune system health is significantly impacted by improved sleep quality, which is achieved via practicing relaxation methods, establishing regular sleep schedules, and designing a sleep-friendly atmosphere.

Conclusion

As we conclude our trip through the complexities of the Autoimmune Paleo Protocol (AIP), it is clear that managing autoimmune disorders involves more than simply dietary changes; it involves a whole-life approach. For individuals looking to navigate their wellness path, the pillars of the autoimmune protocol (AIP)—diet, stress management, sleep, exercise, and knowledge of the intricacies of autoimmune health—form a complete framework.

AIP is a way of thinking that emphasizes internal healing above external healing. It's not merely a food plan. The creation of an atmosphere that promotes the body's natural ability for balance and healing, gives people the power to take control of their health.

The cornerstones of treating autoimmune disorders include knowing how diet affects inflammation, how important stress management is for immune control, and how important restorative sleep is. Finding harmony means striking a careful balance between taking care of the body, mind, and body's natural healing abilities.

As you go on your road, never forget that progress is a process. Even little actions toward health add up to great accomplishments. Accept every step, acknowledge your accomplishments, and develop a resilient, self-compassionate mentality.

I hope that this information will help you in your journey to resilience, energy, and a balanced existence. Accept the knowledge you have learned and set off on your path to wellness with newfound energy, knowing that every decision you make that is in line with your health and happiness will bring you one step closer to your ideal state of health.

Week 1-4:

Day 1-7 (Repeat for 4 weeks):

- **Breakfast:**
  - AIP Blueberry Muffins with Coconut Yogurt
- **Lunch:**
  - AIP Chicken Salad Lettuce Wraps
- **Dinner:**
  - AIP Carrot Ginger Soup with Grilled Chicken

Week 5-8:

Day 1-7 (Repeat for 4 weeks):

- **Breakfast:**
  - AIP Pumpkin Spice Porridge with Coconut Milk
- **Lunch:**
  - AIP Turkey and Avocado Wrap (using lettuce leaves)
- **Dinner:**
  - AIP Zucchini Noodles with Meatballs

Week 9-12:

Day 1-7 (Repeat for 4 weeks):

- **Breakfast:**
  - AIP Sweet Potato Toast with Avocado
- **Lunch:**
  - AIP Tuna Salad with Mixed Greens

- **Dinner:**
  - AIP Lemon Herb Roasted Chicken with Steamed Broccoli

Week 13-16:

Day 1-7 (Repeat for 4 weeks):

- **Breakfast:**
  - AIP Breakfast Sausage Patties with Sautéed Spinach
- **Lunch:**
  - AIP Turkey and Sweet Potato Hash
- **Dinner:**
  - AIP Baked Salmon with Roasted Brussels Sprouts

Week 17-20:

Day 1-7 (Repeat for 4 weeks):

- **Breakfast:**
  - AIP Plantain Pancakes with Berries
- **Lunch:**
  - AIP Chicken and Vegetable Stir-fry
- **Dinner:**
  - AIP Beef Stew with Root Vegetables

Week 21-24:

Day 1-7 (Repeat for 4 weeks):

- **Breakfast:**
  - AIP Banana Coconut Smoothie

- **Lunch:**
  - AIP Shrimp Salad with Mango Dressing
- **Dinner:**
  - AIP Turkey Meatloaf with Mashed Cauliflower

Week 25-28:

Day 1-7 (Repeat for 4 weeks):

- **Breakfast:**
  - AIP Cinnamon Apple Cereal with Coconut Milk
- **Lunch:**
  - AIP Egg Salad Lettuce Wraps
- **Dinner:**
  - AIP Garlic Herb Roasted Pork Tenderloin with Asparagus

Week 29-32:

Day 1-7 (Repeat for 4 weeks):

- **Breakfast:**
  - AIP Mixed Berry Chia Pudding
- **Lunch:**
  - AIP Shrimp and Avocado Salad
- **Dinner:**
  - AIP Turkey Cutlets with Roasted Squash

Week 33-36:

Day 1-7 (Repeat for 4 weeks):

- **Breakfast:**

  - AIP Spinach and Mushroom Omelette

- **Lunch:**

  - AIP Turkey Bacon Wrapped Asparagus

- **Dinner:**

  - AIP Balsamic Glazed Chicken Thighs with Cauliflower Rice

Week 37-40:

Day 1-7 (Repeat for 4 weeks):

- **Breakfast:**

  - AIP Pear and Cinnamon Breakfast Bowl

- **Lunch:**

  - AIP Eggplant and Beef Casserole

- **Dinner:**

  - AIP Herb Crusted Roast Beef with Green Beans

Week 41-44:

Day 1-7 (Repeat for 4 weeks):

- **Breakfast:**

  - AIP Kiwi Coconut Smoothie

- **Lunch:**

  - AIP Chicken and Cabbage Stir-fry

- **Dinner:**

  - AIP Lamb Chops with Roasted Root Vegetables

Week 45-48:

Day 1-7 (Repeat for 4 weeks):

- **Breakfast:**
    - AIP Orange Ginger Smoothie
- **Lunch:**
    - AIP Turkey Stuffed Bell Peppers
- **Dinner:**
    - AIP Pork Tenderloin with Braised Kale

Week 49-50:

Day 1-7 (Repeat for 4 weeks):

- **Breakfast:**
    - AIP Strawberry Basil Breakfast Salad
- **Lunch:**
    - AIP Chicken and Zucchini Skewers
- **Dinner:**
    - AIP Beef and Broccoli Stir-fry with Cauliflower Rice